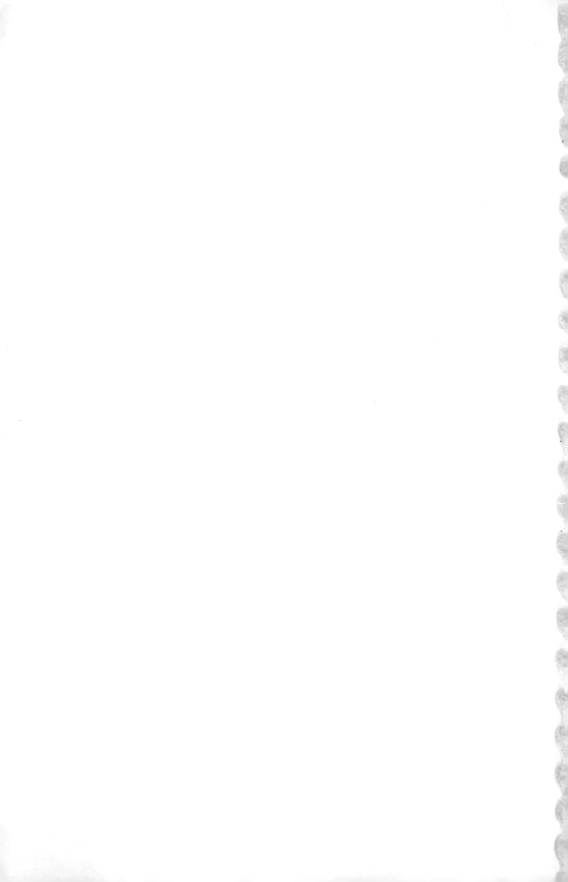

Research in Criminology

Series Editors
Alfred Blumstein
David P. Farrington

Research in Criminology

The Social Ecology of Crime

Edited by
James M. Byrne
Robert J. Sampson

Springer-Verlag New York Berlin Heidelberg
London Paris Tokyo

James M. Byrne
Department of Criminal Justice,
Center for Criminal Justice Research, University of Lowell,
Lowell, Massachusetts 01854, U.S.A.

Robert J. Sampson
Department of Sociology, University of Illinois, Urbana,
Illinois 61801, U.S.A.

Series Editors
Alfred Blumstein
Department of Public Affairs, Carnegie-Mellon University,
Pittsburgh, Pennsylvania 15213, U.S.A.

David P. Farrington
Institute of Criminology, University of Cambridge, Cambridge,
CB3 9DT, United Kingdom

With 6 Figures

Library of Congress Cataloging in Publication Data
Main entry under title:
The Social ecology of crime.
   (Research in criminology)
   Bibliography: p.
   Includes index.
   1. Crime and criminals—United States—Addresses,
essays, lectures. 2. Human ecology—United States—
Addresses, essays, lectures. I. Byrne, James M.
II. Sampson, Robert J.   III. Series.
HV6789.S62   1986   364.042′0973   85-27823

The use of general descriptive names, trade names, trademarks, etc. in this publication, even
if the former are not especially identified, is not to be taken as a sign that such names, as
understood by the Trade Marks and Merchandise Marks Act, may accordingly be used
freely by anyone.

Typeset by Ampersand Publisher Services, Inc., Rutland, Vermont.
Printed and bound by R. R. Donnelley and Sons, Harrisonburg, Virginia.
Printed in the United States of America.

9 8 7 6 5 4 3 2 1

ISBN 0-387-96231-X Springer-Verlag New York Berlin Heidelberg
ISBN 3-540-96231-X Springer-Verlag Berlin Heidelberg New York

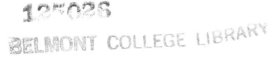

Preface

In this volume we present a series of research papers broadly concerned with the social ecology of crime and delinquency. The theme is the search for the underlying social causes of phenomena such as criminal victimization, delinquency, violent and property crime, neighborhood fear, neighborhood deterioration, and recidivism. We have selected research by authors who are concerned with *both* social-structural (e.g., age, sex, race, and family composition) and ecological (e.g., size, density, crowding, etc.) characteristics of aggregates (e.g., neighborhoods, cities) as important units of analysis in their own right. We also include studies which attempt to measure the contextual effects of aggregate characteristics on individual behavior. The authors of these chapters have raised— and attempted to answer—a number of intriguing questions about neighborhoods, cities, and crime:

1. Does analysis of previously ignored elements of neighborhood structure (such as family disruption and guardianship factors) improve our understanding of why some neighborhoods have higher rates of personal criminal *victimization* than others?
2. Which theoretical model of the *fear* of crime—victimization, social control, or economic viability—is supported by an analysis of interneighborhood variation in levels of fear?
3. Do delinquency rates actually *accelerate* ongoing patterns of neighborhood transition, indicating that there is a reciprocal relationship between delinquency rates and ecological change?
4. Why do some cities have higher rates of crime and other forms of "unconventionality" (e.g., conflict, suicide) than others? Are these differences due to ecological or nonecological factors?
5. What has been the impact of the dramatic changes in demographic composition (age, sex, race) of the largest U.S. cities on crime trends between 1960 and 1980?
6. Which causal model of crime—cultural or structural—offers the better explanation of intermetropolitan and regional variation in violent crime rates?

7. By considering the *socioenvironmental context* into which an offender is released after a period of incarceration, can we improve upon recidivism predictions which are based solely on personal characteristics of the offender?
8. Does the apparent relationship between gun ownership and violent crime vary by sex of owner and/or type of gun? And, more importantly, does gun ownership have an *independent* effect on the rate of violent crime once elements of the community structure (e.g., density, poverty, family disorganization, urbanization) are introduced into the analysis?

We believe that answers to the above questions will provide important insights into the nature of the relationship between community context and crime. Despite differences in methodological approach across studies, the papers we have selected for inclusion in this volume share a common focus on the macrosociological or structural determinants of crime and its consequences (e.g., fear, neighborhood disorganization, ecological change).

By focusing on the *social* context of crime, the present volume differs from many recent publications in the area of *environmental* criminology that have devoted much attention to "spatial" concerns. For example, several recent books (e.g., Harries, 1980; Brantingham and Brantingham, 1981, 1984; Hakim et al., 1982; Georges-Abeyie and Harries, 1980) include discussion and analysis of such issues as the directions that offenders travel to commit crimes, the distance they travel, the mapping of crime and victimization patterns, and other geographical concerns. While research on the geography of crime is no doubt important, with roots in the early ecological analyses of Shaw and McKay, it can and should be distinguished from the social ecological perspective.

Berry and Kasarda (1977, p. 10) have observed that an intrinsic feature of contemporary ecological inquiry is that it is predominantly macrosocial in perspective. Indeed, a "fundamental assumption of the ecological approach is that social systems exist as entities 'sui generis' and exhibit structural properties that can be examined apart from the personal characteristics of their individual members" (Berry and Kasarda, 1977, p. 13). Consequently, we believe that there are community structural effects on crime that are independent of (and causally prior to) individual effects. Although criminologists are perhaps further from the realization of the social ecological paradigm than other more established subfields such as urban sociology (for an overview see Micklin and Choldin, 1984), the empirical research in the present volume demonstrates that progress is being made.

We begin our presentation in Chapter 1 with an analysis and discussion of several key issues in the social ecology of crime including a brief overview of the historical context of ecological inquiry. We then divide our presentation of research papers into three sections. In Part I, Neighborhood Level Analyses of Crime, Victimization, and Fear, we have included three papers at the intraurban level of analysis. In Part II, Interurban Analyses of Violent and Property Crime, we have selected three papers which use cities, SMSAs, and regions as the units of analysis. In Part III, The Impact of Ecological Factors on Decision making and Policy in the Criminal Justice System, we have included two papers which analyze criminal justice policy areas—parole release and gun control—from a social ecological perspective. Taken together, the chapters which follow provide a comprehensive presentation of social ecological perspective on the causes and consequences of crime, victimization, and fear.

Contents

Contributors

David J. Bordua Department of Sociology, University of Illinois, Urbana, Illinois 61801, U.S.A.

Robert J. Bursik, Jr. Department of Sociology, University of Oklahoma, Norman, Oklahoma 73069, U.S.A.

James M. Byrne Department of Criminal Justice, Center for Criminal Justice Research, University of Lowell, Lowell, Massachusetts 01854, U.S.A.

Roland Chilton Department of Sociology, University of Massachusetts, Amherst, Massachusetts 01003, U.S.A.

Stephen D. Gottfredson Department of Criminal Justice, Temple University, Philadelphia, Pennsylvania 19122, U.S.A.

Stephanie W. Greenberg Strategic Planning, Mountain Bell Telephone Company, Denver, Colorado 80202, U.S.A.

Richard Rosenfeld Department of Sociology, Skidmore College, Saratoga Springs, New York 12866, U.S.A.

Robert J. Sampson Department of Sociology, University of Illinois, Urbana, Illinois 61801, U.S.A.

Ralph B. Taylor Department of Criminal Justice, Temple University, Philadelphia, Pennsylvania 19122, U.S.A.

1
Key Issues in the Social Ecology of Crime

JAMES M. BYRNE AND ROBERT J. SAMPSON

In this opening chapter, we highlight six key issues that are of concern to both researchers and theorists interested in the community context of crime: (1) The data source controversy; (2) the question of theory integration; (3) the problem of contextual fallacies; (4) conceptualization and measurement issues in ecological research; (5) the use of cross-sectional versus longitudinal designs; and (6) the applications of social ecology to public policy.[1] In each of the following eight chapters, one or more of these issues is empirically addressed. However, before assessing these issues, we feel it will be helpful to briefly place the ecological study of crime in its historical perspective. The obvious centerpiece for such an inquiry is the work of Shaw and McKay and the recent expansions, reformulations, and "rediscoveries" of their basic propositions.

Shaw and McKay Revisited

Much of contemporary criminological theory can be traced to the seminal ecological studies of Shaw and McKay conducted at the University of Chicago in the 1920s and 1930s.[2] Indeed, Baldwin and

---

[1]These issues have been identified and discussed in recent reviews of ecological research. See for example Bursik (1984), Sampson (1983a), Dunn (1980), and Baldwin (1979) for reviews of neighborhood-level research; and Byrne (1983), Brantingham and Brantingham (1981), and Harries (1980) for reviews of city-level research on crime.

[2]The history of the social ecology of crime can be traced back further than Shaw and McKay. Pioneering ecological efforts by the 19th century French sociologists Quetelet and Guerry constituted some of the first work in "scientific criminology" according to Vold (1958, p. 164). Other Europeans, such as Rawson and Mayhew, also figured prominently in development of the ecological perspective. For an interesting review of the origins and development of English ecology and its relationship to American criminology, see Morris (1957).

Bottoms (1976) have observed that this is not only true of the cultural transmission theory but also of the differential association theory of Edwin Sutherland and Thorsten Sellin's culture conflict perspective. Unfortunately, a complete review of the Shaw and McKay tradition is beyond the scope of this introductory chapter.[3] Because of the importance of the work of Shaw and McKay, however, we provide a brief overview of their community ecological framework and its pervasive influence on later intra- and interurban studies of crime and delinquency. We also examine recent trends in research on the social ecology of crime and the extent, if any, to which they bear on the Shaw-McKay framework.

Clifford Shaw (1929) was one of the first American sociological researchers to demonstrate the marked variations of delinquency rates within a major city. Shaw and his later associate McKay (1931) showed that the highest delinquency rates in Chicago were located in deteriorated zones in transition next to the central business and industrial district. Rates of delinquency were found to decrease as distance from the center of the city increased, except in areas characterized by industry and commerce. These findings led Shaw and McKay to conclude that delinquent behavior was closely related to the growth processes of the city as outlined by Park (1916) and Burgess (1925). In areas characterized by the disintegrative forces of industrialization, the community ceased to be an effective agency of social control. Delinquency areas were specifically characterized by low economic status, heterogeneity, and mobility (see Kornhauser, 1978).

In their later work, Shaw and McKay (1942) investigated further the relationship between the social systems of neighborhoods and the growth processes of the larger city. In particular, they attempted to account for their earlier finding that high rates of delinquency persisted in certain areas over many years, independent of population turnover. Shaw and McKay (1942, p. 320) argued that delinquent and criminal patterns of behavior were transmitted socially in areas of social disorganization. Autonomous, delinquent subcultures were hypothesized to have arisen in socially disorganized communities and perpetuated through a process of cultural transmission, where traditions were passed down through generations. Shaw and McKay also presented data from Philadelphia, Richmond, Cleveland, Birmingham, Seattle, and Denver that indicated the same patterns of persistent delinquency as Chicago.

---

[3]Excellent reviews of the Shaw and McKay tradition have been provided by Pfohl (1985), Bursik (1984), and Finestone (1976). The critique of early ecological research by Baldwin and Bottoms (1976) is also informative.

Intracity and Intercity Research on the Social Ecology of Crime

Many of the ecological studies conducted as an outgrowth of the Shaw-McKay model concentrated on one variable: economic status. This is not surprising, since Shaw and McKay considered poverty to be the most important determinant of variations in delinquency rates. Three oft-cited studies (Bordua, 1958; Chilton, 1964; Lander, 1954) specifically examined the independent effects of economic status on delinquency. Although economic status was generally inversely related to delinquency in all three studies, the independent effects in multivariate analysis were inconsistent. In particular, Lander (1954) and Bordua (1958) both argued that once factors such as home ownership were controlled, the effects of poverty on delinquency were weak. However, Gordon (1967) has criticized the work of Lander and argues that once proper statistical techniques are introduced, poverty is a strong predictor of delinquency.

Most intraurban studies demonstrate a positive bivariate relationship between poverty and crime but like the Lander-Bordua-Chilton studies, there is ambiguity regarding the strength of the effect in multivariate analysis.[4] For this reason, summarization of the literature regarding the preponderance of evidence suggests that "the probability of occurrence of a complex of acts collectively called 'crime' is relatively high in low status areas." Similarly, Kornhauser's review of the literature leads her to comment that the "ecological correlation between community economic level and delinquency rate is high and secure" (1978, p. 100). Despite such assessments, the causal status of poverty as an ecological determinant of crime and delinquency continues to be debated (see, e.g., Baldwin, 1979; Braithwaite, 1979; Sampson & Castellano, 1982).

In addition to economic status, neighborhood-level research has generally documented a positive relationship between crime/delinquency and the following community characteristics: percent nonwhite, proportion of youthful males, crowded housing, mobility, and structural density. It should be emphasized that this summary pertains to bivariate correlates of crime and delinquency. As with economic status, the assessment of multivariate effects is not straightforward because of collinearity among ecological variables and differences across studies regarding methodology, units of analysis, and crime types. Still, recent reviews of the ecological literature (Baldwin, 1979; Dunn, 1980; Harries,

---

[4]A number of researchers have demonstrated a positive relationship between poverty and crime but yielded inconsistent patterns regarding partial effects or failed to perform multivariate analysis. See Harries (1980) or Baldwin (1979) for a complete review.

1980; Kornhauser, 1978) tend to conclude that poverty and racial composition are the most consistent and strongest predictors of crime and delinquency rates within cities. These findings obviously buttress the Shaw and McKay tradition.

A recent review of *intercity* (and inter-SMSA) research by Byrne (1983) reaches similar conclusions about the social ecology of crime and delinquency using this broader unit of analysis.[5] City-level research has generally linked crime and delinquency to a variety of physical characteristics (e.g., density, overcrowding, city size, population change, division of labor, ecological position, and opportunity) and/or aggregate characteristics of the resident population (ethnicity, age composition, occupational/employment diversity, economic factors [e.g., income, poverty, inequality], family composition, education, citizenship, and gender). Unfortunately, any assessment of the magnitude of these relationships and the relative importance of these variables is somewhat misleading, for intercity (interurban and inter-SMSA) analyses conducted during the past 20 years have varied along a number of critical dimensions.

1. Different data sources were used (i.e., UCR, Victimization).
2. Different types of analysis were conducted (i.e., bivariate, multivariate) which were limited by a variety of factors (e.g., multicollinearity).
3. Different units of analysis were employed (i.e., city, urbanized area, SMSA).
4. Sample size varied greatly and when cities were used, minimum city size varied (e.g., from population 4,000 to 100,000 and up).
5. Different research designs were employed (i.e., cross-sectional and longitudinal).
6. The number and type of predictor and criterion variables differed from study to study.
7. Different measures of key explanatory variables were used (Byrne, 1983).

In summary, it is apparent that ecological researchers have not ignored either the neighborhood or the city as an object of study. These researchers have often tried to adapt the theoretical perspective of Shaw and McKay to their examinations of intra- and intercity variations in both property and violent crime. The results of their research have at once underscored the importance of the ecological paradigm and the need to broaden its theoretical focus (Baldwin & Bottoms, 1976).

---

[5]Harries (1980) includes a similar summary of the available evidence on cities and crime that also highlights a set of geographical factors not discussed here, including, for example, climate, seasonality, and phases of the moon.

The Changing Focus of Social Ecology

It is in this context that a number of recent changes in the scope (and methods) of ecological research should be noted. For example, one distinct trend in intraurban ecological research over the last few decades has been the use of social area analysis as originally formulated by Shevky and Bell (1955). The theoretical basis of Shevky and Bell's work was the concept of *social* differentiation, as opposed to the earlier Chicago school emphasis on *spatial* differentiation. Shevky and Bell attempted to relate the internal structure of cities to social changes taking place in the wider society, rather than focusing primarily on the ecological processes operating within cities, as did Park (1916) and Burgess (1925).

Shevky and Bell (1955) developed three constructs that they argued were indicative of aspects of the increasing scale of modern, urban industrial society: social rank, urbanization, and segregation. Criminologists have utilized social-area analysis by correlating these constructs with indices of crime in an attempt to delineate the ways in which social structure affects the patterning of crime across ecological areas.[6]

Despite its well-documented limitations (in particular, see the review in Baldwin, 1974), we feel social-area analysis has produced a number of important studies (notably Dunn, 1974; Polk, 1967; and Quinney, 1964). But perhaps the most enduring contribution social-area analysts have offered is the viewpoint that social structure has consequences for crime that transcend geographical space. In this respect, social-area analysis has played an important role in turning the focus of areal research from a strict analysis of geographical and spatial influences to an examination of the social structural determinants of crime. Many contemporary ecological studies have incorporated this viewpoint.

A number of other recent trends in intracity and intercity ecological research can be identified: (1) an attempt by researchers to incorporate explicit measures of area family disruption (e.g., percent divorced/separated and percent female-headed families with children) in the study of crime[7] (Sampson, 1985); (2) a focus on the criminogenic characteristics of the physical environment[8] (based largely on the work of Newman,

---

[6]For example, see Polk's studies of San Diego (1957) and Portland (1967), and Quinney's study of Lexington (1964).

[7]Although many investigators have focused on what Shevky and Bell (1955) termed "family status," this dimension pertains mostly to life-cycle stages such as fertility, female-labor-force participation, and single-family housing (e.g., Quinney, 1964). Measures of family disruption, in contrast, would include percent divorced, percent separated, and percent female-headed households.

[8]For an excellent review of the available research on defensible space theory, see Charles Murray, "The Physical Environment and Community Control of Crime," in Wilson (1983, pp.107-122) and Taylor and Gottfredson (1983).

1972); (3) the inclusion of variables measuring the ecological position of cities, in recognition of the simple fact that criminal opportunities are not a direct function of a city's resident population alone[9]; and (4) preliminary attempts to study intracategory variation in the ecological correlates of crime, in recognition of potential aggregation bias (in particular, see Shichor, Decker, & O'Brien, 1979, 1980).

In summary, there is obviously a continuing line of research in the Shaw and McKay tradition. Our brief overview of neighborhood- and city/SMSA-based research has identified a wide variety of ecological correlates of crime and delinquency. As Shaw and McKay might have predicted, the areal characteristic that has generated the most empirical interest has been socioeconomic status. Indeed, the notion that poverty is an important determinant of crime is deep-rooted in criminological theory (see Blau & Blau, 1982). A second ecological variable that has drawn wide attention is racial composition. Numerous intra- and interurban studies have documented a positive relationship between percent nonwhite and crime and delinquency, a finding that Shaw and McKay would link to the socially disorganized communities in which nonwhites reside. While other structural characteristics have been examined,[10] the disentanglement of the effects of racial composition and poverty/inequality seems to be the major focus of current research on the social ecology of crime.

The relationship between racial composition, economic situation, and crime is also at the core of an important criticism of the social disorganization perspective—the relative inattention to social stratification.[11] Pfohl (1985) recently observed that:

The emphasis on deviance as a natural by-product of rapid social change has led critics to suggest that the disorganization perspective fails to consider the potential causative influence of *structured differences* in social power and social class . . . Research by the Chicago school discovered the highest rates of officially

---

[9]See Gibbs and Erickson (1976), Stafford and Gibbs (1980). The ecological position of a city can be examined by identifying its potential attraction (as reflected by the SMSA/city population size ratio) and its actual attraction (as reflected by its "dominance" of the corresponding SMSA; i.e., city/SMSA retail sales).

[10]For example: overcrowding, population (and structural) density, mobility, age composition, residential stability, neighborhood deterioration, and family disorganization.

[11]See Pfohl (1985, pp. 168-169) for a discussion of this issue. Other criticisms of the social-disorganization perspective are also discussed by Pfohl, including inadequate operationalization of the concept of disorganization confusion of disorganization and differential organization, and the neglect of organized "respectable" deviance.

recorded deviance in the so-called transition zone. This ecological region was said to be most disorganized by social change. Deviance was its unfortunate by-product. Its residents were conceived of as victims of change. Perhaps. But isn't it just as plausible to suggest that its residents were victims of a highly unequal system of social stratification? (p. 168)

However, Pfohl (1985, p. 169) correctly points out that Shaw and McKay recognized the importance of structural factors in their later research on neighborhoods and crime.[12] Indeed, Albert Reiss (1976) has suggested that "one of the great contributions of Shaw and McKay is [the demonstration] that delinquency is endemic in certain neighborhoods and that the problem of becoming delinquent is greater for persons in lower than higher income status groups" (p. 71, as quoted in Pfohl, 1985:169). It appears that the structural critique has been addressed by researchers studying the social ecology of crime, a point we will return to later.

The Data Source Controversy

There are two basic sources of crime data that are used in macro-environmental research: official records collected by either the FBI's Uniform Crime Reporting (UCR) system or by local courts and police agencies, and data collected from victimization surveys. The vast majority of ecological studies have used officially recorded data to generate estimates of crime rates. Criticisms of the UCR are by now well established in the literature (see Hindelang, 1974; Savitz, 1970; Skogan, 1975, for an overview). One aspect of official data has particular relevance when considering the areal analysis of UCR rates. As O'Brien (1983) has recently commented on the Blaus' study (1982), the use of UCR data is questionable when making comparisons across police jurisdictions. While many acknowledge that the UCR underestimates the absolute level of crime, differences in recording and patrol practices across jurisdictions may also affect *relative* comparisons (see also Skogan, 1975).

The advent of victimization surveys in the 1970s provided some answers to the questions raised by critics of official data. Indeed, victimization data are collected independent of the selection mechanisms of the criminal justice system and thus provide a rich data base in which to explore the effects of ecological characteristics on crime. A number of investigators (Decker, 1977; Decker et al., 1982; Nelson, 1979; O'Brien, 1983) have generated estimates of crime rates from the National Crime Survey (NCS) of 26 central cities in the mid-1970s. The NCS-derived

---

[12]This clarification is offered by Finestone and Reiss in their articles in Short (1976) on the Shaw and McKay tradition.

crime rates were then compared with UCR-generated crime rates for the same cities for equivalent crime types. With respect to violent crimes (assault, rape), the preliminary evidence suggests that the UCR and NCS are measuring different phenomena. For example, O'Brien (1983, p. 435) reports that the correlation between UCR and NCS measures of aggravated assault is *negative* (−.36). Cities with a high rate of officially recorded assault as measured by the UCR tend to have low rates of victim-reported assault. The correlation between UCR and NCS measures of rape is trivial (.13). On the other hand, the correlation between theft and property crimes was high (.76 for robbery), providing some evidence of convergent validity.

Although the findings for the 26-city comparison are provocative, they have serious limitations. First, the UCR-NCS comparisons reported by O'Brien (1983) and others were based on a nonrandom sample of only 26 cities, a small number of observations. Second, there are problems with the measurement of assault and other violent crimes in victimization data (see Hindelang, 1978). In particular, blacks and lower-income persons tend to underreport violent crimes to survey interviewers. Thus, the fact that crimes such as assault fail to overlap with UCR rates is not that surprising. What is comforting to the analyst is that robbery and other theft crimes show similar patterns in both NCS and UCR, at least for cities. In any case, it is clear that much additional research is needed at other levels of aggregation to assess the compatibility of offical and victimization data.

We have included papers in this volume using both official and victimization data, at different levels of analysis. The studies by Sampson and Greenberg (Chapters 2 and 3, respectively) employ victimization data; the remaining studies use a variety of official data sources, including arrest data (Chilton, Chapter 6), reported crime data (Byrne and Rosenfeld, Chapters 5 and 7, respectively), juvenile court referrals (Bursik, Chapter 4), and FBI rap sheets (Gottfredson and Taylor, Chapter 8). To the extent that disparate measures of crime produced similar findings despite methodological differences, we have increased confidence in the validity and generalization of results. Thus, by selecting studies employing a wide spectrum of crime measures and units of analysis, we hope to further the development of a general social-ecological perspective.

One final element of the data source controversy can also be highlighted at this point. The problem of accurately defining the population at risk is one faced by researchers using rates based on either official UCR data or victimization survey data.[13] In both instances, the

---

[13]A complete discussion of this issue is found in Byrne (1983, p. 66–71). The potential use of opportunity-specific crime rates has been reviewed in Harries (1981), Sparks (1981), and Gibbs (1978).

population at risk (i.e., the denominator of the crime rate) has been inaccurately limited to city residents; however, while official crime rates include in the numerator crimes perpetuated against residents and nonresidents, victimization surveys include only the victimization of residents. Consequently, as Stafford and Gibbs (1980) have stressed:

Since nonresidents "inflate" the official crime rate of a city, the victimization rates exceed official rates even more than it appears, but the amount of divergence depends, in part, on the ecological position of the city. To the extent that the city has a high population ratio (SMSA/city) and high dominance, the divergence of official crime rates and victimization rates tend to be reduced artificially. (p. 663)

If Stafford and Gibbs are correct, studies that purport to compare official crime statistics with victimization survey data must first control for differences in the ecological position of the cities included in their analyses. (The comparative studies cited earlier did not include this factor in their analyses.)

In his study of the ecological correlates of property crime in U.S. cities, Byrne (Chapter 5) uses both measures of ecological position identified by Stafford and Gibbs (1980). He is thus able to examine the relative importance of this factor in an analysis of intercity variation in the rate of property crime. Not surprisingly, his analysis reveals crime-specific variation in the significance of a city's ecological position. At a minimum, continued attention to factors affecting criminal opportunity is in order, a fact that has been largely ignored by social ecologists.[14]

Is Theory Integration Necessary?

A number of papers in this volume present and analyze "integrated" theoretical models of fear, victimization, and crime. In each case, the authors have attempted to emphasize the convergent aspects of apparently divergent perspectives.[15] For example, Greenberg (Chapter 3) attempts to explain why the fear of crime is so much higher in some neighborhoods than in others. She identifies three alternative theoretical perspectives concerning the fear of crime: a victimization model, a social-

---

[14]There are some notable exceptions, such as the criminal-opportunity perspective (Cohen, 1981; Cohen & Felson, 1979; Cohen, Kluegel, & Land, 1981). See also the observations of Harries (1981) on the development of opportunity-specific crime rates.

[15]A full discussion of the three theory-integration strategies (side-by-side, end-to-end, and up-and-down) critiqued by Hirschi (1979) is beyond the scope of this chapter. Parenthetically, Greenberg (chapter 3) seems to be using an end-to-end strategy, while the other researchers employ variations of the side-by-side strategy. See also Short (1979) for a discussion of the problem of theory integration at different levels of analysis.

control model, and an economic-viability model. The first model hypothesizes that fear will increase with the objective risk of victimization; the second model predicts greater fear in neighborhoods marked by a deterioration of social control; and the third model presents fear of crime as the product of the residents' "sense of confidence in the present and future well-being of the neighborhood." Greenberg's integrated synthesis is provocative, but her findings pose a serious challenge to the social-control model of fear. This underscores a point made by Hirschi (1979): What starts out as theory integration invariably ends up with the rejection of one or more alternative perspectives.

Chapter 5, by Byrne, examines two apparently divergent perspectives on the impact of city life on residents: ecological theory, which offers an urban alienation thesis (see Fischer, 1981, for a review of the Wirthian hypothesis) as an explanation for the higher levels of conflict and crime in larger rather than smaller cities, and the nonecological perspective, which rejects the notion that cities have these effects. Nonecological (or compositional) theorists argue that the physical characteristics of cities will have no independent effects on crime, once we control for the characteristics of city residents. Byrne attempts to integrate the ecological and nonecological perspectives into a general ecological model consistent with the "ecological complex" of Duncan and Schnore (1959) that Bursik (Chapter 4) also uses to study the dynamics of urban change. Focusing primarily on the effect of two elements of the ecological complex (person and environment) on the intercity variation in four property crimes (robbery, burglary, larceny, motor vehicle theft), Byrne finds mixed support for an "integrated" theoretical model, especially when larger and smaller cities are analyzed separately. Nonetheless, he concludes that since neither the ecological nor the nonecological perspective alone can offer an adequate explanation for his findings, we should continue our search for broader explanations.

While both Greenberg and Byrne have attempted to develop and test integrated models, other studies included in this volume were designed to test the competing claims of two or more divergent perspectives. In this sense, they appear to share Hirschi's view that separate and unequal is better and that "a 'successful' integration would destroy the healthy competition among ideas that has made the field of delinquency one of the most interesting and exciting fields in some time" (1979, p. 37).This "competitive" strategy is most often employed in criminology to assess the conflicting claims of strain (e.g., relative deprivation) and subcultural (e.g., subculture of violence) theories concerning the effects of poverty/ inequality and racial composition on crime rates. Since it is clear that these two perspectives dominate theorizing in the social ecology of crime (especially by those interested in intercity variation in crime), the evidence supporting their claims bears close scrutiny.

A number of recent studies have demonstrated a strong effect of percent black on urban crime rates, regardless of poverty and inequality (e.g., Carroll & Jackson, 1983; Messner, 1982, 1983). It has been suggested (see, e.g., Messner, 1983) that these findings support the subculture-of-violence thesis proposed by Wolfgang and Ferracuti (1967) and Curtis (1975). According to Wolfgang and Ferracuti, blacks in urban ghettoes have over time developed a subcultural value system that condones the use of violence. Curtis maintains that the black subculture, which emphasizes physical toughness and exploitation, is an adaptation to the patterns of racial oppression and economic marginality found in the ghetto.

Other investigators (e.g., Blau & Blau, 1982; Loftin & Hill, 1974) have rejected the subcultural model and have argued instead that structural factors account for the positive association between percent black and crime rates. Invoking a relative deprivation theory, Blau and Blau (1982, p. 119) argue that ascriptive socioeconomic inequalities create latent animosities that foster criminal violence. In this viewpoint, percent black is positively related to violence not because of cultural values, but because of structurally rooted forms of racial inequalities in income. In support of their interpretation, Blau and Blau found that economic inequality raised metropolitan crime rates, net of racial composition and regional location.

Not surprisingly, the discrepant nature of these recent findings has generated a lively debate on the validity of subcultural and relative deprivation theories. Two chapters in this volume will illuminate this exchange. In Chapter 7, Richard Rosenfeld tests the competing claims of these perspectives. His conclusion that there is "strong support" for the cultural model directly challenges Blau and Blau's relative deprivation theory. Rosenfeld finds that racial composition is a strong predictor of crime rates regardless of inequality and poverty.

However, in Chapter 2, Sampson observes that much of the research in this debate focuses on the relative importance of racial and economic factors. Consequently, other dimensions of community structure such as social integration and criminal opportunities have been neglected. Sampson's analysis indicates that such factors as family disruption (e.g., percent divorced), residential mobility, and structural density tend to have stronger effects on rates of personal victimization than racial composition and income inequality. He concludes that the disproportionate emphasis on economic and racial factors by subcultural and relative deprivation theorists is misguided.

While the four chapters just highlighted offer no definitive support for simple individual (single theory) or complex mixed (integrated theory) explanations, it should be clear that research on the social ecology of crime is moving toward consideration of a broader range of ecological factors (e.g., opportunity and social integration). In this regard, Ritzer's (1975) discussion of paradigm development in sociology seems pertinent.

We need to spend less time attacking adversaries and more time examining their positions. We might then begin to understand how we can use insights from other paradigms and in the process develop a more unified perspective. (p. 227)

While this approach does *not* preclude dismissal of unsupported theoretical positions, it does suggest that researchers must empirically evaluate alternative explanations comparatively (Elliott, Ageton, & Canter, 1979).

The Problem of Contextual Fallacies

Kornhauser (1978) has posed a difficult and painful question to ecological researchers:

How do we know that area differences in delinquency rates result from the aggregate characteristics of communities rather than the characteristics of individuals selectively aggregated into communities? How do we even know that there are any differences at all once their differing composition is taken into account? (p. 104)

Kornhauser's question is extremely important, for while most ecological researchers infer aggregate-level effects, no controls are introduced for possible confounding individual-level effects. For example, while delinquency may be related to residential mobility of an area, we have no assurance that this relationship would persist if individual mobility were taken into account. If it did not, the effect of aggregate mobility represents individual-level processes rather than the influence of environmental context.

Unfortunately, few studies have been conducted in criminology within a contextual framework. This is not for a complete lack of effort or insight, however. Data on *both* individual and aggregate characteristics across a sample of areas that vary on key variables are difficult to obtain. Most contextual studies have utilized self-reported delinquency data and have been largely concerned with one issue—the relative effects of aggregate and individual socioeconomic status (SES) (see, e.g., Clark & Wenniger, 1962; Johnstone, 1978; Reiss & Rhodes, 1961). Official arrest data across jurisdictions usually do not contain detailed individual-level characteristics, such as income and education, and thus have been unable to address contextual questions. Since self-report data generally yield information confined predominantly to minor infractions, and then only for juveniles, evidence regarding contextual effects of ecological characteristics on homicide, robbery, burglary, and other serious crime is quite limited. Perhaps more important, prior self-report delinquency research has not rigorously explored the contextual effects of community characteristics other than poverty. To a considerable degree, then, the contextual question in the social ecology of crime remains very much alive.

Chapter 8, by Stephen Gottfredson and Ralph Taylor, highlights this issue. They argue that socioenvironmental context affects delinquency rates and postrelease adjustment independent of individual risk factors. Consequently, they analyze the effect of neighborhood context on recidivism, controlling for a number of individual-level characteristics known to predict recidivism (e.g., prior record, age, marital status). In a similar vein, Greenberg (Chapter 3) proposes a model that clearly rests on the assumption that neighborhood characteristics are important in understanding fear of crime above and beyond individual factors that contribute to a sense of vulnerability. To test this model, she explicitly controls such individual characteristics as age, race, sex, and income. In short, by anticipating and controlling for possible individual-level confounding effects, both of the above studies should advance the utility of the social ecological perspective.

Conceptualization and Measurement Issues

Blalock (1982) has observed that:

Conceptualization refers to the theoretical process by which we move from ideas or constructs to suggesting appropriate research operations, whereas *measurement* refers to the linkage process between these physical operations on the one hand, and a mathematical language on the other. The complete process involves a triple linkage among theoretical constructs, physical measurement operations, and mathematical symbols and operations. (p. 12)

There are a number of well-documented problems related to the conceptualization and measurement of the explanatory variables used by social ecologists.[16] We begin with a discussion of conceptualization issues.

A major "conceptual" limitation of ecological research is the decided lack of attention paid to the processes that mediate the effect of community characteristics. Most ecological studies examine the effects of census characteristics on crime or delinquency rates and then infer support for a particular theoretical framework, even though there is no

---

[16]Perhaps the most comprehensive review of this issue is provided by Blalock (1982); See also Langbein and Lichtman (1978). Strategies for addressing problems related to both conceptualization and measurement (e.g., triangulation, confirmatory factor analysis, etc.) are identified by these authors.

empirical evidence demonstrating the presumed mediating process. As Kornhauser (1978) notes:

> ... most delinquency theories take as their point of departure the *same* "independent variables." Age, sex, race, ethnicity, socioeconomic status, size of community—these are the staples of delinquency theory. Even if securely established, the correlation of any or all of these with delinquency is compatible with all extant theories. Consider socioeconomic status. Its correlation with delinquency is assumed by strain models, many control models, and most cultural deviance models. It is the variables that *intervene* between socioeconomic status and delinquency that are at issue. (p. 82)

Indeed, to adequately test a theory it is necessary to empirically establish the relation to delinquency of the interpretive variables it implies (Kornhauser, 1978, p. 82). Thus, the relationship between crime and, for example, percent black does not in and of itself support any one theory.

This general problem is illustrated by the claims of Blau and Blau (1982) stemming from their analysis of SMSA crime rates and census data.

> High rates of criminal violence are apparently the price of racial and economic inequalities. In a society founded on the principle that "all men are created equal," economic inequalities rooted in ascribed positions violate the spirit of democracy and are likely to create deprivation ... The social process that may be inferred is that much inequality engenders alienation, despair, and pent-up aggression, which finds expression in frequent conflicts, including a high incidence of criminal violence. (p. 119)

Note that the Blaus' assertions arise from conjecture, not from direct empirical evidence. That is, the mediating processes of "alienation," "despair," and "pent-up aggression" are inferred from the correlation of aggregate offense rates with census characteristics (notably racial income inequality) of SMSAs. Parallel to the case for individual delinquency, many theoretical scenarios are consistent with an effect of inequality or poverty on crime. It is not until concepts such as disorganization and alienation are measured that the theoretical framework of the Blaus (relative deprivation) is ultimately vindicated. Unfortunately, most ecological researchers share the same dilemma and unwittingly or not are seduced into making strong theoretical claims on the basis of weak or irrelevant evidence.

Indeed, the articles in this volume do not escape completely unscathed from this criticism. No doubt, this is due to the inherent difficulties in designing and collecting measures of intervening constructs across a sample of ecological areas. Not surprisingly, then, most of the studies in this volume discuss ways in which this important area should be addressed in future research.[17]

There are also a variety of measurement issues that can be raised. For example, Byrne (1983) has pointed out that even a cursory review of the empirical research on cities and crime reveals that not only the *number* of variables employed but also the *measures* of these variables vary from study to study, making a simple summary of findings misleading. Thomas Orsagh (1979) identified one aspect of this problem: We have multiple indicators of key explanatory variables. In certain instances, the selection of indicators will affect the results of the study. Indeed, Orsagh suggested that:

> While empirical research can err from want of an appropriate statistical proxy for the theoretical construct at issue, it can also flounder from having too many proxies from which to choose. (p. 288)

To illustrate his point, Orsagh reviewed the literature on the effect of economic status on crime and quickly identified seven measures of legitimate income and five unique indicators of employment opportunity. He concluded that:

> This plethora of possibilities makes the difficult task of comparative analysis well-nigh impossible. [For example] How can one explain the failure of empirical research to discover a statistically significant relation between employment opportunity and crime when the appraisal of the results of that research seemingly requires a comparison of apples and oranges? (1979, p. 288)

While the "apples/oranges" analogy is ultimately an empirical question, few researchers have explored the practical and theoretical implications of the selection of key explanatory variables. The implicit assumption is that we are simply dealing with alternative measures of the same theoretical construct. But is this true? For example, Laub (1980, p. 29) observed that the use of multiple indicators of urbanism has resulted

---

[17]In the meantime, Blalock (1982) offers an approach to this measurement problem that bears consideration: "The only constructive stance that I can suggest is one that admits to the nature of the problem, distinguishes between those theoretically defined variables that have and have not been associated with operational measures, attempts to state explicitly the assumptions required to link the former theoretical constructs with their indicators, and then proceeds to specify just which propositions can and cannot be tested with the data at hand." (p. 20) See Blalock (1982: Chapters 1 & 2) for a more detailed explanation. According to Blalock, "This stance basically admits that data collection constraints will mean that certain important variables cannot be measured, but it retains these variables in the model as unmeasured variables and thus permits the statement of a number of theoretical propositions that themselves cannot be tested with the data"(p. 20).

in confusion regarding not only the measurement but the meaning of this concept.

The diversity of the measures of key ecological variables is not limited to employment opportunity and urbanism. What is the appropriate measure of income? The percentage of families below the poverty line (Sampson, Castellano, & Laub, 1981)? the median family-income (Beasley & Antunes, 1974; Harries, 1976; Quinney, 1966; Schuessler, 1962; Stafford & Gibbs, 1980)? the median income of males in the experienced civilian labor-force? What is the most accurate measure of age composition? The percentage of males 15-24 (Avio & Clark, 1976)? the percent of youth 15-30 (Stahura, Huff, & Smith, 1978)? the percentage of population 18 and over (Myers, 1980)? the percentage of the population 15-35 (Schuessler, 1962)? Clearly, the selection of indicators is not a simple, straightforward process. For this reason, the comparison of findings based on different measures of key variables may often be ambiguous.[18]

However, it is not the *diversity* of measures per se that is problematic for ecological researchers; It is that certain predictor variables may be inadequately measured. For example, Roncek argues that aggregation bias is inherent in most city-level density measures (e.g., population per square mile) and that "the percentage of high-density neighborhoods or the percentage of persons living in high-density areas is the correct index to use" (1975, p. 846). In addition, Stokols advocates the development of a crowding measure that looks at its spatial component but also is sensitive to its experiential qualities, "in which the restricted aspects of limited space are perceived by the individuals exposed to them" (1972, p. 275). Inadequate measurement has been a problem associated with other variables as well, including ethnicity, inequality, family composition, and opportunity.[19] Thus, the question can legitimately be raised: Are we measuring what we *think* we are measuring? Recognizing this problem, we have included papers that offer an excellent compendium of some of

[18]Indeed, this is the starting point for many debates over the relative merits of apparently divergent perspectives on the causes of crime and delinquency. When "inconsistent" findings are reported, advocates of the challenged perspective often point to inadequate measurement of explanatory variables as the "cause" of the discrepancy. This point is underscored in the recent debate over the age/crime relationship highlighted in the *American Journal of Sociology* between Greenberg (1985) and Hirschi and Gottfredson (1985).

[19]For a discussion of measurement problems related to each of these variables, see the following sources: on ethnicity (Chilton, 1985; Chilton & Sutton, 1986); on inequality (Blau & Blau, 1982; Rosenfeld, Chapter 7, this volume); on family composition/disruption (Cohen, 1981; Harries, 1980; Sampson, chapter 2, this volume); on opportunity (Cohen, 1981; Cohen & Felson, 1979; Byrne, chapter 5, this volume).

the best available measures of these variables at the intra- and interurban level of analysis.

The Use of Cross-Sectional Versus Longitudinal Designs

By far the vast majority of ecological studies have examined the relative effects of structural characteristics on crime in cross-sectional analysis at one point in time.[20] This is somewhat ironic given that classic ecological theory is concerned with processes of change in urban areas. From the early works of Park, Burgess, and Shaw and McKay to the more recent work of Duncan and Schnore (1959), Hawley (1971), and Berry and Kasarda (1977), ecological inquiry has had a strong interest in the dynamics of change in neighborhoods and cities. Recognizing the extent to which this mandate is linked to the ecological paradigm, Bursik and Webb (1982) tackled the issues of community change and crime. Using longitudinal data from 1940, 1950, and 1960, Bursik and Webb (1982) found that since 1950 changing neighborhoods tend to be characterized by changing levels of delinquency. That is, changing neighborhood composition was associated with higher levels of delinquency for the period 1950 through 1960. However, there are precious few studies in the criminological literature that have advanced a dynamic perspective of the effects of community characteristics on criminality. If we are to maintain the rich tradition of ecological inquiry that has been set in other subfields of sociology, researchers must attempt to gain leverage on the study of communities over time. This is no easy task; for as the bulk of ecological research in criminology might indicate, the data available for such a task are rare and difficult to obtain.

Chapter 4, by Robert Bursik, and Chapter 6, by Roland Chilton, offer two unique perspectives on the dynamics of community change. Bursik draws on the ecological complex of Duncan and Schnore (1959) to examine the general process of urban change. He is primarily interested in the effect of crime (an indicator of community disorganization) on the characteristics of urban neighborhoods in Chicago and whether "crime rates have themselves accelerated or altered the ongoing processes of community change." Clearly, Bursik is challenging the "typical" ecolo-

---

[20]See the critique of this approach in ecological research by Bursik (1984). Byrne (1983) identifies the three basic advantages of the cross-sectional design: (1) a more refined unit of analysis is possible; (2) more units of observation can be examined; and (3) a wider range of predictor variables can be utilized. An interesting debate on the relative merits of longitudinal versus cross-sectional research is provided by Greenberg (1985) and Hirschi and Gottfredson (1985).

gist's assumption that ecological variables (and ecological change) affect crime rates (and not vice versa). His analysis reveals that delinquency rates are not only one of the *outcomes* of urban change; they are an important part of the *process* of urban change itself. Perhaps most significantly, Bursik observes that "although changes in racial composition cause increases in the delinquency rate, this effect is not nearly as great as the effect that increases in the delinquency rate have on minority groups being stranded in the community." He notes that this finding seems to be consistent with Shaw and McKay's original description of the dynamic process of urban change.

One surprising finding that emerged from Bursik's analysis is that while socioeconomic status (SES) is not related to delinquency, high rates of delinquency were followed by significant gains in the SES of the neighborhood. Bursik speculates that the recent "gentrification" process occurring in many large U.S. cities has fundamentally changed the relationship between SES and delinquency. It appears that crime is only one of a number of factors (including, e.g., housing costs and values, racial composition, etc.) that the new urban "settlers" evaluate when choosing a place to live. Finally, Bursik underscores the fact that the change process occurring in American cities is dynamic and as such cannot be adequately examined using a cross-sectional design.

The second dynamic analysis included in the current volume is by Chilton (Chapter 6). Arrest and census data for twelve of the largest cities in the United States were examined by Chilton to assess the relative importance of changes in age, gender, and racial composition for increases in arrests from 1960 to 1980. He concludes that it is the changing racial composition of these large cities that has the greatest impact on arrest counts. Specifically, arrest rates for cities increased rather dramatically from 1960 to 1980; in large measure this is due to increases of the black population of central cities. Interestingly, this phenomenon occurs even though black male arrest rates remained stable over the same time periods. As Chilton observes, the large increase stems from the higher prevalence of "black offending" than "white offending," in conjunction with the absolute increase in the size of the black population. (Interestingly, racial composition is related to crime [and victimization] at both the neighborhood city and SMSA level, according to the research presented in this volume.[21])

Chilton speculates that this recent trend may be due to the "relative deprivation" and the socialization of our nonwhite urban population. "Among the most plausible interpretations of this trend are the persis-

---

[21]See the Chapters 2, 4, 5, and 7 in this volume by Sampson, Bursik, Byrne, and Rosenfeld respectively.

tently limited economic circumstances of young nonwhite men and women and the changing family arrangements of those remaining in large areas of many central cities." As we observed earlier, the importance of family ties is substantiated (at the neighborhood level) by Sampson's analysis. However, the relative deprivation perspective is challenged by both Sampson and Rosenfeld (Chapters 2 and 7, respectively, this volume).

Finally, Chilton's research also improves our understanding of age composition and crime while directly challenging (1) the recent assertion by Hirschi and Gottfredson that "the age-crime relation is invariant across sex and race" (1983, p. 556), and (2) Greenberg's assertion that there is a single juvenile class.[22] Given the current debate concerning the proper interpretation of the age-crime relationship, these conclusions take on added significance.

The Application of Social Ecology to Criminal-Justice Policy

There are a variety of ethical, legal, and political issues related to the application of ecological research to decision-making in the criminal-justice arena. To begin, there is clearly a debate over the proper role of social scientists in social-policy discussions. It is somewhat ironic to observe that the early ecological researchers from the Chicago School have been identified simultaneously as *objective social scientists* who infused scientific methods into a largely *un*scientific discipline (Pfohl, 1985) and as the *classic social reformers* of the past 50+ years, who participated in one of the most important community-change experiments of the 20th century (Baldwin & Bottoms, 1976).[23] While early Chicago sociologists such as Robert Park, in fact, have attempted "to dissociate themselves from the image of sociology as social reform" (Pfohl, 1985, p. 155), the legacy of Shaw and McKay's Chicago Area Project was the strategy of social control through community organiza-

---

[22]See the original articles by Hirschi and Gottfredson (1983) and Greenberg (1979), as well as the subsequent commentary by Chilton (1985), Greenberg (1985), and Hirschi and Gottfredson (1985).

[23]On the other hand, Robert Park, for example, has offered that, "It is probably not the business of the universities to agitate reforms nor to attempt directly to influence public opinion in regard to current issues. To do this is to relax its critical attitude, lessen its authority in matters of fact"(1967, xi, as quoted in Pfohl, 1985, p. 155). Nonetheless, Baldwin and Bottoms point out that "in the history of 'urban criminology' prescriptions for social action have not been lacking"(1976, p. 191).

tion rather than individual change.[24] Subsequent community-level social-control strategies have been based on the assumption that the social ecology of neighborhoods and cities does affect individual behavior. Although we take no position on the proper role of social ecologists in creating changes in "community context," we will highlight the implications of the new body of research presented in this volume for social policy generally and criminal justice policy in particular.

An excellent example of the application of ecological research to decision making in the criminal-justice system is found in Chapter 8 by Stephen Gottfredson and Ralph Taylor. The authors found that the "risk" of recidivism posed by parolees relased into 90 Baltimore neighborhoods was explained (at least in part) by a set of previously overlooked socioenvironmental variables, including such factors as level of incivility, deterioration of the neighborhood, and other situational factors. Monahan (1981) suggested the usefulness of differentiating higher- and lower-risk environments.

Ideally, it eventually might be possible to make differential predictions of the sort that individuals with dispositional characteristics of type N would have X probability of violent behavior if they resided in environment type A, and Y probability if they resided in environment type B. (p. 132)

Other potential applications of Gottfredson and Taylor's person-environment interaction model include pretrial-release and community-sentencing decisions.[25] Of course, the possible utilization of information regarding neighborhood context in making such decisions raises legal, ethical, and practical issues that cannot be (and are not) sidestepped by the authors.

David Bordua's concluding paper (chapter 9) provides a second illustration of how a broader focus on social ecology can shed light on current policy concerns, in this case gun-control policy. It is commonly assumed, for example, that gun availability increases violent crime. Indeed, in a recent influential paper, Cook (1983, p. 51) flatly states: "I believe that the widespread availability of firesarms has a profound influence on violent crime patterns " Bordua's analysis takes issue with

---

[24]This observation is made by Pfohl (1985, p. 155). Schlossman and Sedlak (1983) provide an excellent examination of the early years of the Chicago Area Project (CAP). In addition, see the interviews with Solomon Kobrin and other colleagues of Shaw and McKay at CAP, including Anthony Sorrentino, Joseph Puntil, and Yale Levin in Laub (1983, pp. 87-105; 235-260). A somewhat different view is provided by Snodgrass (1976).

[25]A variety of other police, court, and correctional decision-making applications for these data can be found in Byrne (1984).

this claim in two respects. First, by disaggregating the rate of firearms ownership by both sex of owner and type of gun, Bordua demonstrates that male gun ownership is essentially unrelated to the violent-crime rate in 101 Illinois communities (once important structural characteristics are controlled). Perhaps more interesting, the rate of female ownership is *inversely* related to the violent-crime rate. But rather than simply concluding that guns reduce crime, an inference dictated by conceptualizing gun ownership strictly as an exogenous variable, Bordua posits a model in which gun ownership is a *response* to violence and fear among females. In other words, it appears that communities characterized by high density, urbanization, family disorganization, and poverty generate high rates of violent crime, which in turn produce high levels of fear among women; subsequently, these women turn to gun ownership for protection. The negative relationship of female gun ownership and crime is apparently the complex result of larger community processes that can only be captured by studying the context of community change over a period of time.

Bordua's chapter is thus consistent with Bursik's analysis (chapter 4) in suggesting that crime itself may be considered an exogenous social-ecological variable. In any event, while the findings, of course, call for replication in other contexts, the implication is that to the extent current gun-control legislation is enacted without full consideration of the ramifications of social-ecological processes, it may be seriously misguided.[26]

The remaining authors also discuss the implications of their research for policy. For example, consider Greenberg's analysis (chapter 3) of why the fear of crime is so much higher in some neighborhoods than in others. She concludes that "strategies aimed at fear reduction primarily through fostering contacts among neighbors may be less than optimal." Instead, she recommends that we do two things, in the following order: (1) strenghten the economic well-being of, and sense of confidence in, neighborhoods to reduce fear; and (2) reduce victimization to reduce fear.

On a different issue, Rosenfeld's analysis (chapter 7) revealed that "cultural" variables (e.g., racial composition) offered the best explanation for inter-SMSA variation in violent crime rates, suggesting that we should *not* expect strategies aimed at reducing poverty and inequality to reduce these rates. Other strategies, perhaps aimed at reducing the opportunity for violence by refining the situational context (e.g., controlling the availability of alcohol, guns, and drugs)[27] or changing family, peer, or

---

[26]Walker (1985, pp. 149-164) provides a cogent summary of the relative merits of liberal and conservative gun-control policies, including a critical review of the research on guns and crime.

community values would be preferable. As a counterpoint to Rosenfeld, both Chilton (chapter 6) and Sampson (chapter 2) present a slightly different perspective on the causes of (and solution to) this problem. Indeed, Chilton concludes "that the economic situation of millions of nonwhite men and women is one of the best explanations for increases in crime and arrests" in our nation's largest cities, while Sampson cautions that the implications [of ecological research] for public policy are not straightforward. Byrne (chapter 5) offers a similar caveat when discussing the social policy implications of his research on property crime.

Finally, Bursik's analysis (chapter 4) forces us to consider the race-crime relationship from yet another perspective: "Although changes in racial composition cause increases in the delinquency rate, this effect is not nearly as great as the effect that increases in the delinquency rate have on minority groups being stranded in a community" This finding is interesting, but we must also consider the potential confounding influence of the "gentrification" process.[28] Bursik hypothesizes "that potential 'gentrifiers' may be attracted to nonminority neighborhoods characterized by single-family dwelling units in areas of high de-linquency" due to the cost of housing in low-crime nonminority areas. If Bursik's hypothesis is correct, then perhaps it is the "relative" economic viability of a neighborhood, given its racial composition, that helps explain *both* the pattern of gentrification and lower levels of fear in some high-crime neighborhoods. In any event, it is apparent that further inquiry into the nature of the relation between delinquency and ecological context is in order.

In summary, we should point out that the research presented in this volume represents only a starting point with regard to the potential policy implications of research focused on the community context of crime, victimization, and fear. There are many more fruitful lines of inquiry that we suspect will open in the near future. Thus, it is the purpose of this volume to present a broad agenda for theory, research, and policy on the social ecology of crime. This agenda will take shape in the chapters that follow.

---

[27]See, for example, the approach advocated by Mark Moore (in Wilson, ed., 1983, chapter 8) or the discussion of the major situational correlates of violent behavior in Monahan. (1981, pp. 132-136)

[28]Indeed, Bursik (1984) points out that Schuerman and Kobrin (1983) present findings for Los Angeles that are not consistent with these results.

Part I Neighborhood Level
Analyses of Crime,
Victimization, and Fear

2
Neighborhood Family Structure and the Risk of Personal Victimization

ROBERT J. SAMPSON

Income inequality is the cornerstone of sociological theories focusing on strain and relative deprivation (see Blau & Blau, 1982; Rosenfeld, Chapter 7, this volume). Not surprisingly, then, a great deal of contemporary ecological research has focused on the relationship between community economic factors and crime. In particular, a recurrent issue addressed in recent articles has been the relative effects of economic inequality and racial composition on urban crime-rates (especially Bailey, 1984; Blau & Blau, 1982; Messner, 1982, 1983; Williams, 1984; Rosenfeld, Chapter 7, this volume).

While the social class question is an important one, its dominance in guiding ecological inquiry has tended to shift attention away from family structure as a source of variation in crime rates. I argue that family dissolution has important macrolevel consequences for both informal and formal social control in the community. Also, I review the thesis of Felson and Cohen (1980), who argue that the extent of primary (e.g., single) individual households has important consequences for effective guardianship, and hence for criminal opportunities. Unfortunately, these notions have not been systematically addressed in the research literature, especially at the local community and neighborhood level. This is potentially a serious limitation since community family structure is related to racial and socioeconomic factors (Sampson, 1985), suggesting that many recent studies have been misspecified. For instance, both percent black and poverty are positively related to rates of divorce/separation and female-headed families. There is a strong possibility, then, that casual inferences attributed to race and poverty are in fact due to underlying patterns of family disruption, an issue which has not been fully explored.

To address these and other imbalances in recent research, this chapter extends the focus of the social ecology of crime to explicitly include aspects of neighborhood family structure relating to social control and guardianship. In particular, the goal is to examine the independent effects of divorce and separation, female-headed families, and primary individual households on the risk of personal victimization.

The data base is the national sample of the National Crime Survey (NCS) for the years 1973-1975. Victimization data are collected independent of the selection mechanisms of the criminal justice system and thus provide a rich data base in which to explore the effects of neighborhood characteristics on crime. This is an important advantage since by far the vast majority of prior ecological studies have used officially-recorded crime records (e.g., Uniform Crime Reports) to generate estimates of crime rates. As many have observed (e.g., O'Brien, 1983), the use of official data may be problematic when making comparisons across police jurisdictions. For example, differences in recording and arrest practices may affect even the relative comparison of crime rates across areas.

Victimization data alleviate the official bias problem and thus provide an alternative window from which to view the crime process in relation to community characteristics. Limited ecological research has been conducted with the city sample of the NCS surveys (see e.g., Decker, Shichor, & O'Brien, 1982), but as noted in Chapter 1, this body of research has serious limitations. For example, the NCS city sample was based on a nonrandom selection of only 26 cities. Moreover, the city data pertain to a high level of aggregation and do not necessarily reflect on neighborhood processes that foster crime. The neighborhood was the unit of analysis for some of the classical early literature in ecology and crime (e.g., Bordua, 1958; Chilton, 1964; Lander, 1954; Shaw & McKay, 1942). Since then, however, relatively little has been done at the neighborhood or community-level of analysis, primarily because of data limitations arising from the collection and interpretation of police records. In the present study I attempt to shed new light on the impact of neighborhood influences on crime by studying the extent to which family structure predicts the risk of personal victimization.

Theoretical Framework

Family disruption is theoretically important from a community perspective for several reasons. First, neighborhoods with pronounced family disruption are in all likelihood less able to provide an effective network of formal social controls. Formal social controls may be attenuated since communities with high family dissolution tend to suffer low rates of participation in formal voluntary organizations and local affairs (cf. Kasarda & Janowitz, 1974; Kornhauser, 1978; Tomeh, 1964, 1973). Participation is important since formal organizations attempt to integrate individuals with the larger community (Tomeh, 1973: p. 89). In particular, Kornhauser argues (1978: p. 81) that the family has the potential to perform many functions that link youth to institutions, thus providing institutional routes to valued goals. Since married-couple families exhibit higher degrees of participation in formal organizations than divorced and unmarried people (e.g., Tomeh, 1973), it is logical to expect that pronounced family disruption in a community may interfere with the individual and collective efforts of families to link youth to the wider society through institutional means (e.g., school, religion, sports).

Perhaps a more important consequence of family dissolution is attenuated *informal* controls. Examples of informal social control include neighbors taking note of and/or questioning strangers, watching over each others' property, assuming responsibility for supervision of general youth activities, and intervening in local disturbances (see e.g., Greenberg et al. 1984). The informal nature of collective family social-control has not often been studied. Instead the effect of the behavior and supervision of parents has traditionally been studied only on the delinquency of their own children. But children are often supervised, watched, and even reprimanded by those other than their own parents. Skogan (1986: p. 24) notes: "In stable neighborhoods residents supervise the activities of youth, watch over one another's property, and challenge those who seem to be up to no good" (see also Skogan & Maxfield, 1981: p. 105). In a related vein, research on informal group participation has shown that married-couple families have a higher rate of contact with neighbors than divorced and single people (Tomeh, 1964: p. 33). Thus, in areas with a cohesive family structure parents often take on responsibility not just for their own children, but for other youth as well.

Note that the conceptualization proposed here does *not* necessarily require that it is the children of divorced or separated parents that are engaging in crime. Rather, I take a structural perspective and focus on the effects of family disruption in a community on all residents. Youth in stable family areas, regardless of their own family situation, probably have more controls placed on their leisure-time activities, particulary with peer groups. A well-documented fact in delinquency research is that delinquency is a group phenomenon (Zimring, 1981). Hence, neighborhood family structure is likely to be quite important in determining the extent to which neighborhood youth are provided the opportunities to gather with friends free of the supervision or knowledge of adults (cf. Riley, 1985). This conception may help to resolve the apparent paradox concerning the tenuous relationship between delinquency and broken homes at the individual level (Wilkinson, 1980). But the paradox exists only if one conceives of family disruption as a strictly microphenomenon. To the contrary, the available evidence suggests that families and communities are mutually connected, and thus to the extent the former is disrupted, so are certain aspects of community life.

Rather than concentrating simply on the socialization and social control of juveniles, some have argued that family dissolution is also a proxy indicator for overall disorganization and alienation in adult personal relationships. As Blau and Blau (1982: p. 124) argue:

Disproportionate numbers of divorced and separated in a population may be indicative of much instability, disorientation, and conflict in personal relations. Marital breakups entail disruptions of profound and intimate social relations, and they generally occur after serious estrangement, if not prolonged conflict.

Further, since serious crime is largely a male phenomenon, it may be that divorce contributes to a pool of unattached males freed from the social controls introduced by a married lifestyle. Hence, marital and family disruption appear to be relevant for adults as well as juveniles.

Finally, Felson and Cohen (1980; see also Cohen & Felson, 1979) note the important influence of family structure not just on the control of offenders, but on the control of criminal targets and opportunities. Felson and Cohen argue that traditional theories of crime emphasize the criminal motivation of offenders without considering adequately the circumstances in which criminal acts occur. In particular, predatory crime requires the convergence in time and space of offenders, suitable targets, and the absence of effective guardianship. The spatial and temporal structure of routine activities plays an important role in determining the rate at which motivated offenders encounter criminal opportunites. Felson and Cohen (1980) document the importance of family-activity patterns in determining the opportunity structure of predatory criminal behavior. They note that the proportion of primary individual households (e.g., singles, nonrelatives) is an overall indicator of guardianship. Those who live alone (e.g., single women) are more likely to be out alone (e.g., going to work, restaurants, night clubs, etc.) than married persons and are thus more vulnerable to personal crimes (e.g., rape, robbery). Also, leaving the home unguarded during the day (and night) increases the risk of household crimes. Therefore, a community with a high proportion of primary individual households presents a more attractive environment for crime than areas with a strong family orientation.

In support of their theory, Felson and Cohen (1980) demonstrated that independent of factors presumed to reflect the supply of motivated offenders (e.g., unemployment, age composition), primary individual households had a significant and positive effect on crime trends in the U.S. from 1950 to 1972. They concluded that "the convergence in time and space of suitable targets and the absence of capable guardians can lead to large increase in crime rates without any increase or change in the structural conditions that motivate individuals to engage in crime" (Cohen & Felson, 1979: p. 604).

In this chapter I examine whether the percent of primary individuals in a neighborhood exerts an influence on victimization independent of neighborhood family disruption. Based on the theoretical framework developed above, family disruption and guardianship, while related, nonetheless represent conceptually distinct factors and hence are hypothesized to have independent effects on victimization. Specifically, divorce and female-headed families reflect the disruption of family life and are expected to attenuate community social-control, especially of youth. These disruption factors are hypothesized to increase victimization risk independent of guardianship. On the other hand, primary individual households reflect in large part the prevalence of singles (never married) in an area, which is hypothesized to decrease guardianship capacity and hence increase the opportunities for predatory crime. In addition, both neighborhood family dissolution and guardianship are hypothesized to effect victimization rates independent of culture and structural conditions that motivate individuals to engage in crime (e.g., inequality, unemployment, racial composition).

Data and Method

The data base is the National Crime Survey (NCS) national household sample. The data were collected by the United States Bureau of Census, in cooperation with the Bureau of Justice Statistics of the U.S. Department of Justice. The NCS is a continuous panel survey in which nationally representative samples of households and persons are interviewed twice per year, at six-month intervals.[1] Crimes are classified according to definitions used in UCR (see Webster, 1978). This study is concerned with personal crimes of *theft* (robbery and larceny with contact) and *violence* (rape, aggravated assault, and simple assault). The annual interview sample has approximately 60,000 households containing about 136,000 individuals. The data used in this study are from the survey years 1973 to 1975, representing approximately 400,000 interviews with household respondents.

Each household record in the NCS sample contains information on the socio-demographic, economic, and physical characteristics of the neighborhood in which the household was sampled. The data set used in this study was formed by combining households with similar values of neighborhood characteristics according to 1970 census statistics.[2] To

---

[1]For additional details of the NCS design and collection procedures see Garofalo and Hindelang (1977).

[2]To preserve confidentiality, neighborhoods defined by the Census Bureau are not identifiable census tracts, but are aggregated enumeration districts or block groups with a population minimum of 4,000. A study of these neighborhoods indicated that the aggregation procedure utilized by the Census Bureau resulted in neighborhoods being relatively compact, contiguous, and homogeneous areas

construct reliable rates each neighborhood characteristic was classified into categories of low, medium, and high.[3] The NCS national sample was used to estimate both the population base 12 years of age and older (persons under age 12 are not eligible to be interviewed) and the number of victimizations that occurred each year to persons residing in each category or combination of categories of neighborhood characteristics. The neighborhood characteristics and their measures are as follows: *income inequality* (Gini Index of Income Concentration)[4]; *unemployment* (percent unemployed persons 16 years and older); *racial composition* (percent black); *residential mobility* (percent persons 5 years and older living in different houses than 5 year ago); and *structural density* (percent of units in structures of five or more units). Three aspects of neighborhood *family structure* were selected: percent divorced/separated of those ever married, percent female-headed families, and percent primary individual households. The latter refers to household heads living alone or with nonrelatives only.

Analysis of variance models are used to examine the effects of neighborhood characteristics on personal victimization. Analysis of variance is well suited to the structure of the NCS data analyzed in this study, consisting of interval-level measurement of dependent variable (rates of victimization) and grouped categories (low, medium, and high) of the independent variables.[5] The levels of neighborhood characteristics

---

approximately the size of a census tract (U.S. Bureau of Census, undated). Because neighborhood characteristics were derived from the 1970 census, all housing units constructed since then (about 9% of the sample) do not have neighborhood characteristic identifiers, and are thus excluded from analysis.

[3]See Sampson, Castellano & Laub (1981) for a discussion of how cutting points were determined, and for additional details on methodological issues arising from analysis of the neighborhood characteristic data set.

[4]Preliminary analysis also used poverty (percent of families with less than $5,000 income) as an indicator of economic status. However, the results were largely identical to those obtained when the Gini Index was utilized. This is not surprising, since the Gini and poverty are strongly positively related in this study (gamma = .85) and in others (e.g., r = .81 in Rosenfeld, 1982). Inequality is used as the main economic variable because it has received the most theoretical attention in recent years.

[5]Some researchers have used log-linear models to analyze victimization data (see e.g., Cohen, Kleugel, & Land, 1981). However, this data-analytic option was rejected in favor of analysis of variance for several reasons. First, log-linear models apply to the analysis of dichotomous dependent variables, whereas the present study is an analysis of rates measured on an interval scale. Second, the phenomenon of multiple victimization is inconsistent with the victim-nonvictim dichotomy employed in log-linear analysis. Ecological theory predicts that neighborhood characteristics have an effect not just on the prevalence of

are considered in a fixed effects model (see Kleinbaum & Kupper, 1978: p. 246). Based on previous analysis of NCS data, victimization rates are assumed to be a multiplicative function of independent variables and random error (i.e., linear in the log scale; see Nelson, 1978, 1980; Sampson, 1985). The additive effects assumption of ANOVA models is met by taking logarithms of the rates (see e.g., Nelson, 1978; Sampson, 1985). Multiplicative parameters were obtained by taking antilogarithms of the effects.[6]

In the analyses reported below rates of victimization for each combination of levels of neighborhood characteristics were estimated separately for the survey years 1973, 1974, and 1975. For example, the rate of victimization for persons living in a neighborhood with low inequality and a high divorce rate was estimated separately for the sample years 1973 to 1975. In all, then, each cross-classification was estimated three times.[7] The analysis of variance treated each triad of rates as if they were independent observations made under identical conditions. Differences in rates were then used as estimates of random error, thus allowing an assessment of the statistical significance of both main and interaction effects in the ANOVA models.[8]

---

victimization, but also on the incidence of victimization. It is likely, for instance, that in high risk environments some persons suffer repeated victimizations, a possibility that is masked by treating victimization as a dichotomy. Finally, previous ecological research using official data has almost always been based on rates. Thus, given the NCS data structure in conjunction with the desirability of comparing findings with prior research, analysis of variance seems most appropriate to the task.

[6]Elsewhere (Sampson, 1985) I have examined the sensitivity of results to various weighting schemes employed in the analysis of victimization rates (e.g., case weights, cell weights, and an unweighted orthogonal design). In general the results were consistent regardless of weights. In the present study an unweighted design is used except in cases where there were relatively few observations per cell (e.g., three-way ANOVA in Table 2.6), in which case cell weights were employed. In a cell-weighted design the proportion of persons at each combination of levels of the independent variables are used as weights to reflect the unbalanced nature of the data.

[7]Data limitations guided the extent to which neighborhood characteristics were cross-classified. In general, it was not possible to analyze anything greater than a 3-by-3-by-3 array because of sample size. Despite the large number of interviews, higher order classifications produced empty cells because of the interrelationships among neighborhood characteristics and because of the overall low prevalence of victimization experiences.

[8]Note that if only 1 year of data were used to estimate rates there would be only one observation per cell. In this case there is no within-cell sum of squares to use as a measure of random error. With no residual sum of squares one cannot compute an F-ratio to test statistical significance of the model. To assess

It is important to identify and discuss a distinct limitation of the NCS data that bears on the present study: While the census data refer to characteristics of the victim's neighborhood, the NCS survey did not ask precisely where victimizations occurred.[9] Fortunately, research on the spatial dynamics of crime indicates that a large proportion of serious personal crimes (e.g., robbery, rape, aggravated assault) occur near the residences of both victims and offenders (see e.g., Pokorny, 1965; Pyle, 1974; Reiss, 1967). Furthermore, it seems reasonable to assume that victimizations that take place outside the neighborhood boundaries defined by the census occur more frequently in adjacent or nearby neighborhoods than distant neighborhoods. Given the residential segregation patterns dominant in American metropolitan communities (see e.g., Sorensen & Taeuber, 1975), a given neighborhood is likely to be similar to nearby neighborhoods. It is thus not necessary to assume that all victimizations occurred in the victim's neighborhood to study the risk factors posed by neighborhood characteristics. Indeed, a major proposition of recent theories of victimization (Hindelang, Gottfredson, & Garofalo, 1978; Cohen & Felson, 1979) is that *proximity* to offenders and criminogenic areas is a major determinant of victimization risk. Simply living in a certain type of neighborhood increases risk factors that influence probabilistic exposure, even if some victimizations occur outside specific neighborhood boundaries specified by the Census Bureau.

Recent examination of NCS data supports these observations. Sampson, Castellano, and Laub (1981) and Sampson (1983a) compared rates of victimization for a subset of victimizations that occurred at or near the victim's home[10] with total rates of victimization. As expected, the patterns for "at or near home" rates were reflective of total rates for five neighborhood characteristics. In fact, Sampson (1983a) showed that the "at or near home" patterns for structural density were virtually identical

---

statistical significance in this special case of one rate per cell, one typically assumes there is no interaction in the data, and then the interaction sum of squares is substituted for the residual sum of squares (Kleinbaum & Kupper, 1978; Iversen & Norpoth, 1976: pp. 69-70). Unfortunately, this method precludes the analysis of higher-order interactions. In contrast, the method used in this study does not force the investigator to pool interaction terms into the residual sum of squares.

[9]For example, the NCS place of crime category, "on street, park, field," representing about 45% of all victimizations, does not specify the neighborhood of occurrence. One may be victimized in the street in one's own neighborhood or in the street outside of one's neighborhood.

[10]The "at or near home" category includes "at or in own dwelling; in garage or other building on property; yard, sidewalk, driveway, carport, apartment hall." This category represents about 20% of all victimizations.

to total patterns, controlling for extent of urbanization. Given the strong congruence between at home and total rates, it was concluded that although some victimizations undoubtedly take place in settings extraneous to the victim's neighborhood, such events do not offset overall *patterns* of relationships—the ultimate criterion of theoretical interest. Therefore, in the present study rates of victimization were constructed from total personal victimizations.[11]

Findings

I begin analysis by comparing the effects of income inequality and the divorce rate on theft and violent victimization in SMSA central cities. As noted earlier, inequality has been frequently studied in recent ecological research, and is the key construct in relative deprivation theory (see Blau & Blau, 1982; Rosenfeld, Chapter 7, this volume). It is thus of interest to begin with a direct examination of the independent effects of neighborhood marital disruption and inequality. Based on previous research using NCS data (Sampson, Castellano, and Laub, 1981; Sampson & Castellano, 1982) I limit analysis to central cities within metropolitan areas. As shown by Sampson and Castellano (1982), neighborhood economic status and inequality have attenuated effects on victimization in suburban and rural areas, but rather strong effects in urban centers. Table 2.1 thus presents a severe test of the independent effects of divorce since inequality is allowed its full range of explanatory power.

The results in Panel A reveal that inequality and divorce both have significant (p < .01) main effects on theft victimization. Surprisingly, inequality does not have a significant effect on rates of violent personal crime, whereas divorce exhibits an F-ratio greater than seven. Interaction effects are not significant at the .01 level and do not appear to play an important role in predicting victimization.

Although statistical significance is essential in determining relationships it is necessary to explicitly examine the *direction* and *magnitude* of the effect estimates to assess the substantive importance of variables. Hence, Panel B of Table 2.1 presents effect parameter estimates for the two neighborhood characteristics, and also the percent of variance explained by each factor. Using the multiplicative model one can estimate predicted rates for levels of the independent variables. For example, the overall level of theft victimization in central cities (per

---

[11]It is problematic to examine only "at or near home" rates because when neighborhood characteristics are simultaneously considered the large reduction in sample size tends to produce unreliable rates. See Sampson, Castellano, & Laub (1981) for a full discussion of the place of crime occurrence issue.

TABLE 2.1. Analysis of Variance of Personal Criminal Victimization[a] in SMSA Central Cities, by Neighborhood Income Inequality, Percent Divorced/Separated, and Type of Crime,[b] NCS National Data, by Year (1973–1975)

A. ANOVA Statistics

Source of variation	Degrees of freedom	Theft			Violent		
		Mean square	F	Significance	Mean square	F	Significance
Main effects							
1. Income inequality	2	.205	13.4	.00	.009	.4	.67
2. Percent divorced	2	.436	28.4	.00	.192	7.9	.00
Interaction							
12	4	.007	.5	.74	.076	3.1	.04
Residual	18	.015			.024		

B. Parameter Estimates[c]

Type of crime and neighborhood category	Income inequality		Divorced/separated	
	Effect	R^2	Effect	R^2
Theft (Grand $\bar{X}$ = 1662)				
Low	.62		.50	
Medium	1.04	25.8	.65	54.8
High	1.46		1.46	
Violent (Grand $\bar{X}$ = 3147)				
Low	.89		.56	
Medium	1.02	1.7	.88	33.5
High	1.05		1.19	

[a]Estimated rates of victimization were transformed to logarithmic (base 10) scale.
[b]Theft crimes include robbery and larceny. Violent crimes include rape, aggravated assault, and simple assault.
[c]Multiplicative parameters obtained by taking antilogarithms of the effects.

100,000 persons) is 1,662. The effect of living in a neighborhood with a high divorce rate is to raise this rate by a factor of 1.46, yielding a predicted theft rate of 2,426 (1,662 × 1.46). Conversely, the low category of divorce has a predicted rate of 831 (1,662 × .50). Hence, the predicted rate in high divorce areas is almost three times greater than the rate in low divorce areas, independent of the effect of income inequality.[12] Note that this ratio is equivalent to simply taking the ratio of effect parameters (i.e., 1.46/.50 = 2.9). The pattern of effects can thus be easily shown by taking ratios. In addition, Panel B displays estimates of R^2, in this case revealing that divorce alone explains 55% of the variance in personal-theft victimization, compared to 26% for inequality. As for violent crime, inequality explains less than 2% of the variance, whereas divorce accounts for about 34%.

The results to this point are rather clear—neighborhood marital disruption has important effects on rates of both theft and violent victimization. In fact, the effects of divorce were considerabley stronger than the effects of income inequality. The recent emphasis on inequality as a major criminogenic condition thus appears to be at least somewhat misleading. Indeed, in separate analysis of variance models for central cities, percent primary individuals had stronger effects on personal victimization than income inequality, as did racial composition, density, and residential mobility (data not shown in tabular form).

The only economic-related neighborhood characteristic noted by Sampson and Castellano (1982) that had a consistent significant effect on victimization (controlling for individual characteristics) in the total sample of the NCS (i.e., urban, suburban, and rural areas) was the unemployment rate. Thus, to further explore the effect of neighborhood economic structure Table 2.2 presents an analysis of variance of theft and violent victimization in the United States by percent primary-individual households and percent unemployed. Both neighborhood factors have a significant ($p < .01$) effect on rates of theft and violent crime. However, the percent of primary individuals in a neighborhood has a stronger effect on theft victimization ($R^2 = 52$) than unemployment ($R^2 = 30$). This pattern is reversed for the risk of violent victimization, where unemployment explains more than twice the amount of variance than primary

---

[12]The actual value of the overall level of victimization is not of theoretical interest to the present study nor are the actual values of the predicted rates. The overall level is simply a standard against which to compare relative increases and decreases associated with neighborhood effects. The central research question is how neighborhood characteristics influence victimization rates. This question is most easily answered by examining ratios of effect parameters, and by comparing the relative amount of variance in the total sum of squares explained by each characteristic.

TABLE 2.2. Analysis of Variance of Personal Criminal Victimization[a] in SMSA Central Cities, by Neighborhood Unemployment, Percent Primary Individual Households, and Type of Crime,[b] NCS National Data, by Year (1973–1975)

A. ANOVA Statistics

Source of variation	Degrees of freedom	Theft			Violent		
		Mean square	F	Significance	Mean square	F	Significance
Main effects							
1. Unemployment	2	.119	36.27	.00	.044	19.01	.00
2. Primary individuals	2	.204	62.13	.00	.016	6.81	.00
Interaction							
12	4	.019	5.67	.00	.005	2.02	.14
Residual	18	.003			.002		

B. Parameter Estimates[c]

Type of crime and neighborhood category	Unemployment		Primary individuals	
	Effect	R^2	Effect	R^2
Theft (Grand $\bar{X}$ = 1,514)				
Low	.79		.74	
Medium	.95	30.2	.93	51.8
High	1.32		1.44	
Violent (Grand $\bar{X}$ = 3,090)				
Low	.85		.98	
Medium	1.00	49.0	.93	17.6
High	1.17		1.12	

[a] Estimated rates of victimization were transformed to logarithmic (base 10) scale.
[b] Theft crimes include robbery and larceny. Violent crimes include rape, aggravated assault, and simple assault.
[c] Multiplicative parameters obtained by taking antilogarithms of the effects.

individuals. Note also that the interaction of unemployment and primary individuals for theft victimization is significant at the .01 level. This interaction stems from the increased effect of primary individuals on theft victimization for persons residing in medium and high unemployment neighborhoods.

In brief, the results confirm that independent of unemployment levels—which Cohen and Felson (1979) argue are an indicator of the supply of motivated offenders—percent primary individual has significant and rather strong effects on serious personal victimization. In addition, family dissolution (divorce and female-headed families) also has significant positive effects on victimization independent of unemployment (data not shown). The results thus far suggest that neighborhood guardianship and social-control factors both have significant effects on the risk of victimization that are not accounted for by economic factors thought to increase crime (i.e., inequality and unemployment).

An examination of the interrelationships among neighborhood characteristics revealed that racial composition is even more closely related to family structure than economic structure, especially the percentage of female-headed families. For example, the gamma coefficient reflecting the relationship between percent black and percent female-headed families in the U.S. population is .57. This positive and significant coefficient indicates that areas with a large black population also contain a high proportion of female-headed families. Divorce is also positively related to percent black. Therefore, part of the effect of racial composition observed in recent research (e.g., Messner, 1983) may be due to its association with family structure. In a similar vein, it is possible that the effects of family structure in Tables 2.1 and 2.2 may be spurious and due to underlying racial effects. In an attempt to disentangle the effects of race from family structure Table 2.3 presents a simple two-way crime-specific analysis of variance of percent black by percent female-headed families.

First, one notes that the main effect of percent black on violent crime is not significant. Second, even though percent black has a significant effect on theft victimization, the effect of family structure is clearly stronger. For instance, the theft-victimization parameter estimates in Panel B show that the ratio of high/low effect estimates for percent female-headed families is 3.9 compared to 2.9 for percent black. For violent crime, family dissolution explains more variance than percent black by a factor greater than two. Note also that none of the interactions of race and family structure are significant.

The results indicate that family structure has stronger effects on both theft and violent personal-victimization than racial composition. Parenthetically, this result is also supported if we compare the effects of percent divorced separated with racial composition. In this model percent divorced explained 54% of the variance in theft victimization, compared

TABLE 2.3. Analysis of Variance of Personal Criminal Victimization,[a] by Neighborhood Family Structure, Racial Composition, and Type of Crime,[b] NCS National Data, by Year (1973–1975)

A. ANOVA Statistics

Source of variation	Degrees of freedom	Theft			Violent		
		Mean square	F	Significance	Mean square	F	Significance
Main effects							
1. Female-headed fam.	2	.617	35.13	.00	.052	5.37	.01
2. Percent black	2	.327	18.64	.00	.022	2.29	.13
Interaction							
12	4	.002	.14	.96	.002	.25	.90
Residual	18	.017			.009		

B. Parameter Estimates[c]

Type of crime and neighborhood category	Female-headed families		Percent black	
	Effect	R^2	Effect	R^2
Theft (Grand $\bar{X}$ = 874)				
Low	.60		.72	
Medium	.89	55.7	1.08	29.5
High	2.32		2.15	
Violent (Grand $\bar{X}$ = 2558)				
Low	.86		.89	
Medium	.97	31.3	1.09	13.13
High	1.27		1.15	

[a] Estimated rates of victimization were transformed to logarithmic (base 10) scale.
[b] Theft crimes include robbery and larceny. Violent crimes include rape, aggravated assault, and simple assault.
[c] Multiplicative parameters obtained by taking antilogarithms of the effects.

to 35% for percent black (data not shown). For violent victimization percent divorced explained 34% of the variance, whereas percent black explained less than 2%. Thus, regardless of the measure, neighborhood family disruption has much stronger effects on personal victimization than racial composition.

Neighborhood guardianship also has a significant effect on victimization rates independent of race. Table 2.4 reveals that even though percent black exerts significant main effects, percent of primary individuals explains a considerable independent amount of the variation in victimization. Indeed, primary individuals explains 41% of the variance in personal thefts and 56% of the variance in violence. These results, in conjunction with the earlier results, suggest that many of the recent models in ecological research may be misspecified. That is, by failing to incorporate measures of community family-disruption and guardianship, it is possible that large effects attributable to inequality and especially race are in part spurious and due to their association with family structure. Some evidence for this assertion is found in the Blau and Blau (1982) study. Blau and Blau (1982: p. 124) found that percent divorced had greater effect on rates of rape, robbery, and assault than did income inequality or percent black. In fact, both income inequality and racial composition had insignificant effects on rape and robbery when percent divorced was added to the regression model. The Blaus' results are particularly interesting because they are largely consistent with the present study even though SMSAs were employed as units of analysis, a rather large and heterogeneous area.

I noted earlier that neighborhood family structure is theoretically important for several possible reasons. On the one hand, family disruption (divorce among ever married adults; female-headed families) may reduce social controls in the neighborhood. For example, areas with a high proportion of single-parent families, especially with children, may provide fewer constraints and supervision with regard to the activities of local youth (cf. Riley, 1985). Family structure is also important in determining guardianship patterns and hence opportunities for crime. All else equal, areas with a high proportion of primary individual households are vulnerable to predatory personal and household crimes since property is left unguarded and single individuals may be more vulnerable to victimization (cf. Felson & Cohen, 1980). For example, single women are more vulnerable to rape victimization than married women. In essence, then, neighborhood family structure is hypothesized to influence the control of both offenders *and* target opportunities.

If the linkage of routine activity and social-control perspectives is valid, then even though primary individuals and family dissolution are positively related, each dimension should exert an independent effect on rates of victimization. In other words, while areas with a disproportionate number of divorced adults and female-headed families will also contain

TABLE 2.4. Analysis of Variance of Personal Criminal Victimization,[a] by Neighborhood Racial Composition, Percent Primary Individual Households, and Type of Crime,[b] NCS National Data, by Year (1973–1975)

A. ANOVA Statistics

Source of variation	Degrees of freedom	Theft			Violent		
		Mean square	F	Significance	Mean square	F	Significance
Main effects							
1. Percent black	2	.392	207.27	.00	.018	16.42	.00
2. Primary individuals	2	.299	157.78	.00	.042	37.64	.00
Interaction							
12	4	.009	4.82	.01	.002	2.16	.12
Residual	18	.002			.001		

B. Parameter Estimates[c]

Type of crime and neighborhood category	Percent black		Primary individuals	
	Effect	R^2	Effect	R^2
Theft (Grand $\bar{X}$ = 1.096)				
Low	.66		.76	
Medium	.89	53.3	.81	40.9
High	1.70		1.62	
Violent (Grand $\bar{X}$ = 2.692)				
Low	.89		.95	
Medium	1.05	24.0	.89	56.2
High	1.07		1.20	

[a] Estimated rates of victimization were transformed to logarithmic (base 10) scale.
[b] Theft crimes include robbery and larceny. Violent crimes include rape, aggravated assault, and simple assault.
[c] Multiplicative parameters obtained by taking antilogarithms of the effects.

a higher proportion of singles, the two aspects of neighborhood family patterns are theoretically distinguishable. This issue has not been systematically addressed in prior research.

To test the dual effects of neighborhood family patterns I examined the independent effects of both divorce and female-headed families on victimization risk while controlling for guardianship. Table 2.5 presents the results for percent female-headed families. First, note that both dimensions of family structure have significant main effects on personal theft and violent victimization. The parameter estimates in Panel B reveal an interesting type of crime pattern., In particular, theft victimization is predominantly explained by variations in family disruption—female-headed families explain 79% of the variance while primary individuals explain about 17%. On the other hand, the prevalence of primary-individual households does a better job of predicting violence, explaining over half the variance compared to 27% for female-headed families. This pattern is consistent with the theoretical model, for family dissolution (especially female-headed families) is expected to have stronger effects on the social control of juveniles than adults. Since juveniles are more involved in theft crimes than serious violence (i.e. rape, assault) as compared to adults, it is not surprising that female-headed families exert a particularly large effect on theft victimization. On the other hand, areas with a high proportion of singles may provide more rape victims and situations where fights are likely to occur (e.g., bars, social clubs).

As in earlier tables, the pattern of effects for primary individuals is not monotonic—victimization rates are highest in the high category, but the low and medium categories are quite similar with the latter actually showing slightly lower risk factors. For theft victimization, risk factors increase monotonically with increases in the percent of female-headed families, whereas for violent crimes the low and medium categories are essentially identical.

Also, Panel A indicates significant interaction effects for both crime types, much larger than in previous analyses. These effects arise because female-headed families have an increased effect on theft victimization in areas with a large proportion of primary individuals. Similarly, the latter has greater effects on theft victimization in areas with a disproportionate number of female-headed families. The interaction pattern for violent crimes was somewhat inconsistent, indicating mainly that primary individuals had a greater effect in the low categories of intact families. Finally, the results for percent divorced are similar to those shown in Table 2.5. Specifically, if we enter the divorce rate in lieu of female-headed families, both primary individuals and divorce exert independent effects of victimization risk (data not shown). The overall results support the theoretical perspective advanced, and suggest that both vulnerability in target guardianship and attenuated-family social controls are important and independent predictors of victimization.

TABLE 2.5. Analysis of Variance of Personal Criminal Victimization,[a] by Neighborhood Percent Female Headed Families, Percent Primary Individual Households, and Type of Crime,[b] NCS National Data, by Year (1973–1975)

A. ANOVA Statistics

Source of variation	Degrees of freedom	Theft			Violent		
		Mean square	F	Significance	Mean square	F	Significance
Main effects							
1. Female-headed families	2	.508	642.14	.00	.030	77.00	.00
2. Primary individuals	2	.108	136.35	.00	.059	150.92	.00
Interaction							
12	4	.012	15.28	.00	.009	24.03	.00
Residual	18	.001			.000		

B. Parameter Estimates[c]

Type of crime and neighborhood category	Female-headed families		Primary individuals	
	Effect	R^2	Effect	R^2
Theft (Grand $\bar{X}$ = 933)				
Low	.62		.89	
Medium	.89	79.2	.85	16.8
High	1.82		1.35	
Violent (Grand $\bar{X}$ = 2,754)				
Low	.91		.98	
Medium	.93	27.0	.83	53.3
High	1.17		1.20	

[a] Estimated rates of victimization were transformed to logarithmic (base 10) scale.
[b] Theft crimes include robbery and larceny. Violent crimes include rape, aggravated assault, and simple assault.
[c] Multiplicative parameters obtained by taking antilogarithms of the effects.

The final portion of analysis examines the independent effects of marital dissolution and community guardianship when juxtaposed to known determinants of victimization risk. Recent analyses (Sampson, 1985) have established that residential mobility and structural density are two of the most powerful predictors of personal victimization at the neighborhood level. In particular, mobility and density generally have stronger effects on victimization than racial composition, unemployment, economic status, and inequality (see Sampson, 1985). In this chapter as well, family disruption and guardianship have also been shown to predict victimization regardless of racial and economic factors. Hence, as a final test of the explanatory power of neighborhood family structure, Table 2.6 presents a three-way crime-specific ANOVA of the effects of divorce/separation, residential mobility, and structural density on personal victimization.

The results show that the main effects of density, mobility, and divorce are all significant at the .01 level for both theft and violent victimization. However, one notes that divorce has the overall strongest effects, especially for theft crimes. For example, the predicted theft rate in the high category of percent divorced is over *four* times higher than the predicted theft rate in the low category (2.28/.55). The corresponding effect ratios for structural density and mobility are 3.3 and 1.7 respectively. Note also that divorce explains more variance in theft victimization than mobility and density *combined*. When violent crime is the criterion, divorce and mobility have similar effects, each explaining approximately 31% of the variance, while structural density explains about 16%.[13]

A model similar to that in Table 2.6 was estimated in Sampson (1985) where percent female-headed families was analyzed rather than divorce. The results were essentially the same, except that mobility had a slightly greater effect on violent victimization than female-headed families. Finally, I re-estimated the three-way ANOVA in Table 2.6 by entering the indicator of neighborhood guardianship instead of the divorce rate. Despite the significant main effects of mobility and density, primary individual households exerted significant positive main effects on personal victimization (data not shown).

---

[13]The three-way interaction, while significant, does not easily lend itself to interpretation. The theft interaction stems from a larger than expected theft risk in neighborhoods with a high level of structural density and mobility, and a low divorce rate. A disproportionately high violence rate is found in the high density, low mobility, and low divorce category.

TABLE 2.6. Analysis of Variance of Personal Criminal Victimization,[a] by Neighborhood Percent Divorced/Separated, Residential Mobility, Structural Density, and Type of Crime,[b] NCS National Data, by Year (1973–1975)

A. ANOVA Statistics

Source of variation	Degrees of freedom	Theft			Violent		
		Mean square	F	Significance	Mean square	F	Significance
Main effects							
1. Divorced/separated	2	1.58	117.7	.00	.379	84.7	.00
2. Residential mobility	2	.25	18.6	.00	.371	83.0	.00
3. Structural density	2	1.18	88.2	.00	.184	41.2	.00
Interaction							
12	4	.033	.6	.66	.012	2.72	.04
13	4	.008	.6	.68	.002	.55	.69
23	4	.004	.3	.90	.008	1.97	.11
123	8	.044	3.25	.00	.002	4.93	.00
Residual	54	.013			.0045		

B. Parameter Estimates[c]

Type of crime and neighborhood category	Divorced/separated		Mobility		Structural density	
	Effect	R²	Effect	R²	Effect	R²
Theft (Grand X̄ = 827)						
Low	.55		.85		.57	
Medium	.82	44.0	.89	6.9	.84	32.9
High	2.28		1.44		1.91	
Violent (Grand X̄ = 2428)						
Low	.70		.71		.77	
Medium	.95	31.8	.97	31.1	.97	15.5
High	1.44		1.44		1.24	

[a] Estimated rates of victimization were transformed to logarithmic (base 10) scale.
[b] Theft crimes include robbery and larceny. Violent crimes include rape, aggravated assault, and simple assault.
[c] Multiplicative parameters obtained by taking antilogarithms of the effects.

Discussion

The empirical results of the present study demonstrate that whether traditional variables such as race, poverty, and inequality are considered, or more powerful predictors such as mobility and density, neighborhood family structure has significant and substantively important influences on personal criminal victimization. This general result supports the major hypothesis, and underscores the theoretical importance of neighborhood family structure.

The theoretical framework distinguished two dimensions of family structure. First, percent divorced and percent female-headed families were hypothesized to reflect a dimension of marital and family disruption that decreases community social control. In general, both divorce and female-headed families had significant effects on victimization, net of other factors. While there were no explicit measures of informal social control available, the consistency of results lends support to the notion that neighborhoods with a high proportion of family disruption are less able to provide an effective network of social controls. A fruitful area of future research lies in the direct measurement of informal controls (e.g., supervision of youth, watching out for neighbors' property) and explication of the linkages to aspects of community family disorganization.

The second dimension of family structure pertained to guardianship. Relying on the theoretical framework advanced by Felson and Cohen (1980), it was hypothesized that areas with a high proportion of primary individual households would suffer disproportionately high rates of predatory crime. In support of this thesis, primary individual households exerted significant effects on victimization independent not only of racial and economic factors presumed to measure the supply of offenders, but of family disruption (i.e., divorce, female-headed families). The latter result supports the notion that family structure is important with regard to both social control of offenders, and to vulnerability and guardianship factors that influence the opportunities for motivated offenders to carry out criminal acts.

Of course the present results are in no sense definitive. Similar to Felson and Cohen (1980), a proxy for guardianship (primary individual households) was used rather than a direct measure. Future research efforts are thus needed to partition more precisely the effects of social control of offenders from the control of targets and opportunities. For example, areas with high divorce rates may place fewer informal control on potential offenders and also may provide more vulnerable targets of victimization. And as noted by Felson and Cohen (1980: p. 401), "isolated [primary] persons may be less subject to social control and thus more likely to engage in criminal activity. On the other hand, these persons may also be more suitable victims of crimes." But as shown in the present study, *both* family dissolution and primary individual households had significant effects on victimization when simultaneously considered, suggesting that their influences are not redundant.

In sum, the overall results support an integrated model linking a community social-control perspective with the routine activity theory of Cohen and Felson. Clearly, more research is needed before either one of the components of the theory are fully confirmed. But in the meantime, the data suggest that neighborhood family structure should be considered an important community-level factor in explaining victimization risk. Unfortunately, most recent studies have tended to concentrate on racial and economic factors, providing an imcomplete and possible inaccurate picture of community influences on crime.

However, while racial composition and inequality exerted weaker effects than family structure in the present study, that does not imply the former are unimportant and can be ignored. Rather, some have argued that inequality, race, and family disruption are causally linked. For example, one possibility is that racial segregation and economic inequality in black communities lead to pronounced family disruptions, which in turn contributes to increases in crime. One of the advocates of this position is Rainwater (1970), who argues that the pattern of economic inequality and racial oppression which produces and sustains the ghetto is the root cause of marital instability and family breakdown, particularly in the form of female-headed families. In addition, there is an accumulating body of evidence suggesting that the disruption of black families due to racial oppression and the economic marginality of black males has had profound negative implications for black women, particularly for those with children (Rainwater, 1970; Wilson & Neckerman, 1985). In particular, the pool of marriageable (i.e., economically stable) men is proportionally much smaller for black women than white women, thus prolonging periods of financial stress and disruption for black families (Wilson & Neckerman, 1985). In contrast, divorce and separation do not appear to have as long-lasting negative consequences for either financial or family stability in the white population (Bane, 1985). Whites are less likely to be separated than blacks, and more often remarry after divorce (Wilson & Neckerman, 1985). These sorts of models are obviously too complex to be considered here, but are deserving of further research. Indeed, there are a host of questions that remain to be examined regarding the causal linkages among poverty, economic inequality, race, and family disruption.

Acknowledgment: This paper was supported in part by a grant funded by the National Institute of Justice (#81-IJ-CX-0042) entitled "The Neighborhood Context of Criminal Victimization." Points of view expressed herein are those of the author and do not necessarily represent the official position of the Justice Department.

3
Fear and Its Relationship to Crime, Neighborhood Deterioration, and Informal Social Control

STEPHANIE W. GREENBERG

Two important models of the fear of crime have emerged in recent years—the victimization model and the social-control model (Lewis & Salem, 1980, 1981). According to the victimization perspective, a high crime rate leads to a high victimization rate, which leads to a high level of fear in anticipation of being victimized. The social-control model hypothesizes that the deterioration of social control, or the perception that this has occurred, is the source of fear, more than the objective risk of victimization. Several studies have found that the availability of social support or resources to deal with neighborhood problems alleviated fear, particularly in highly threatening residential environments (see e.g., Greenberg, Rohe, & Williams, 1984a; Skogan & Maxfield, 1980; Taub, Taylor & Dunham, 1984). These resources include local networks and community involvement at the individual level, and social cohesion and availability of community organizations at the neighborhood level.

Recent reviews of the literature (Greenberg, Rohe, & Williams, 1984a) indicate support for both models. The evidence suggests that while there may be a direct effect on fear of objective levels of crime or prior victimization, such factors as physical and social vulnerability to crime, vicarious victimization (i.e., hearing about crimes by talking with neighbors), and perceptions of the seriousness of the crime problem have a stronger relationship to fear. With regard to control-related variables, sense of control over and responsibility for the neighborhood on the one hand, and perception of disorder (e.g., vandalism, teens fighting, litter, etc.) on the other, are also correlated with fear, in opposite directions.

No definitive conclusion can be drawn in summarizing past research, however, because few studies have included both crime-related and control-related variables and allowed them to compete against each other. Even more importantly, few studies have included objective measures of crime or social disorganization. In most cases, these factors were measured by subjective perceptions. It is possible that people who are fearful for other reasons may perceive more crime and less control.

There is also a third perspective that has received relatively little attention. It can be termed the economic-viability model, which is concerned with the residents' sense of confidence in the present and future economic well-being of the neighborhood. Taub, Taylor, and Dunham (1984) found that among white homeowners fear had a negative effect on perceptions of the investment potential of the neighborhood only for people who thought the neighborhood was racially unstable and who believed that economic and social decline would result from integration. A hypothesis that can be deduced from this finding is that concern about the economic future of the neighborhood may make individuals feel vulnerable to events that are beyond their control, one of which is crime.

Perceived economic viability and the availability of local sources of social support may be two sides of the same coin—sense of control over one's environment. There may, in fact, be trade-offs between the two. Residents of relatively affluent neighborhoods with strong housing markets and good housing quality may not feel threatened by crime, even when crime rates are relatively high. Confidence in one's investment and in the future of the neighborhood may be an effective buffer against the effects of crime. Residents of low-income neighborhoods are not likely to share this sense of economic security, but the existence of a locally based support network of friends, relatives, and neighbors may help to increase the sense of environmental control.

In the following analysis we examine a synthesis of the victimization, social-control, and economic-viability models of the fear of crime.[1] The model that will guide this analysis is shown in Figure 3.1. According to the model, informal control is an intervening variable between objective neighborhood conditions and fear. Specifically, it is hypothesized that crime level and physical deterioration affect fear directly and indirectly via their effect on perceptions of both the seriousness of the crime problem and social disorder, which in turn affect confidence in the economic viability of the neighborhood and perceived availability of social support. Perceptions that crime and/or disorder are serious local problems are expected to erode confidence in the economic well-being of the neighborhood and to reduce trust in neighbors. Perceived problems related to crime and disorder are expected to affect fear directly as well as indirectly through perceptions of economic viability and helpfulness of neighbors. Individual vulnerability to crime is also expected to affect fear directly and indirectly through its effect on perceived crimes and disorder problems. Physical vulnerability is expressed by age and sex, while social

---

[1]For a detailed empirical and theoretical overview of these three models see Greenberg, Rohe, and Williams (1984a,b).

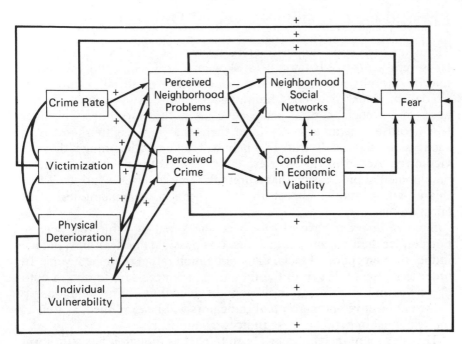

FIGURE 3.1. Conceptual model of neighborhood crime, physical deterioration, neighborhood perceptions, and fear.

vulnerability, that is, exposure to crime by virtue of social position, is expressed by race and economic status.

The Data

The present study is a reanalysis of a data set collected by Richard Taub and associates at the National Opinion Research Center. The data will be described briefly here, but a more detailed description can be found in Taub, Taylor, and Dunham (1984).

The study was conducted in eight neighborhoods in Chicago. Each neighborhood represents one neighborhood in an eight-cell design—a high or low ranking on the reported crime rate, racial change, and property appreciation. The two data-collection efforts that are relevant to the present study are the resident survey and the Housing and Neighborhood Appearance Rating. The Housing and Neighborhood Appearance Rating consisted of a series of ratings of the physical appearance of buildings and surrounding grounds. A 25% random sample of survey respondents was selected. The blocks on which these respondents resided were rated. These data were then attached to the survey file of any respondent who resided on a rated block.

Physical Deterioration, Perceived Disorder, and Fear

There has been considerable interest in the concept of incivilities in the last several years (see Hunter, 1978; Skogan & Maxfield, 1980). Incivilities refer to the physical signs of the deterioration of social control (e.g., vandalism, litter, abandoned buildings, or public drunkenness). Proponents of the social-control perspective argue that incivilities engender fear because individuals infer from them that the neighborhood is in such a state of social disarray that help will not be forthcoming if they are victimized. According to this view, the presence of incivilities signifies a developmental progression that culminates in high levels of crime. While this view has intuitive appeal, there has been no convincing test of its effect on fear.

Signs of disorder have usually been measured by subjective perceptions rather than objective indicators. It is possible that fear may, in fact, induce the perception of social disorganization rather than the reverse. In order to address this gap in the literature, it is necessary to obtain both objective and perceptual indicators of incivilities. The relationship between objective and perceptual indicators will be examined, as well as the relationship between these indicators and fear.

The concept of incivilities has been treated as though it has a uniform effect on perceived social control and fear. There is a need, though, for greater specification of this concept and its effects. Incivilities have typically been measured by asking people which in a list of items is a big problem in the neighborhood. The resulting scores are then combined into an index and used to predict fear, perceived crime level, or the like. Ethnographic research suggests, although does not directly test, that what is fear-provoking in some neighborhoods may not be in others. For example, teens hanging out on a corner may be viewed by the residents of culturally homogeneous, stable, working-class neighborhoods as acceptable and perhaps even positive behavior (Gans, 1962; Spergel, 1964; Suttles, 1968; Whyte, 1955). In such areas, teenage males may be perceived as turf protectors. In neighborhoods where mutual suspicion and hostility prevail (e.g., lower income, heterogeneous, unstable neighborhoods) the same behavior may provoke fear and perhaps avoidance of local hangouts (Merry, 1981a,b). The point is that neighborhoods may have different norms as to what is regarded as acceptable public behavior. The concept of incivilities therefore needs to be broken down into its component parts to examine which have the strongest and most consistent associations with fear and perceptions of social control.

Physical features that were measured at the building or lot level were aggregated into blocks. Indicators of deterioration include housing type (proportion of single-family dwellings, flats, and multiple-unit dwellings on a block), presence or absence of vacant lots, number of abandoned buildings, presence or absence of nonresidential land use, presence or absence of visible signs of housing rehabilitation, number of building flaws (e.g., on roofs, facades, windows, or porches), and amount of trash and litter on lawns and driveways. Perceived disorder was defined by whether each of a series of items was stated to be a big problem or somewhat of a problem in the neighborhood. (See Greenberg, Rohe, & Williams, 1984b: Table A-3.) Five measures of crime perceptions were calculated: (1) belief that there is little or no crime in the neighborhood, (2) belief that the likelihood of being a crime victim in the neighborhood in the next year is low, (3) fear of walking alone in the neighborhood at night, (4) an index called "worry" which included various concerns about crime in the neighborhood,[2] and (5) satisfaction (very satisfied and somewhat satisfied) with safety in the neighborhood).

Relative Effects of Crime, Physical Deterioration, and Informal Social Control on Fear

This analysis examines the relative effects of independent variables that reflect the three perspectives on fear—victimization (crime rate and personal or household victimization), social control (physical deterioration of the neighborhood, perceived disorder, social support networks), and economic viability (confidence in the economic viability of the neighborhood).

Hierarchical stepwise regression was used to predict safety satisfaction and the worry index. Predictor variables were entered in five steps. The first step included objective measures of crime and neighborhood deterioration, followed in order by perceptions of the level of neighborhood crime and other problems, local networks, economic viability of the neighborhood, and a measure of the physical and social vulnerability of the respondent.

Neighborhood crime was defined as the total crime rate per 1,000 population in the census tract in which the respondent resided,[3] and victimization was defined as whether the respondent or a household member had been the victim of one or more crimes in the last year. Physical deterioration was defined by four variables, three of which are factor scores. Eight indicators of physical deterioration were entered into a principal-components factor analysis, with varimax rotation followed

---

[2]"Worry" is a four-item index that expresses relatively vague, nonspecific anxieties about crime, such as feeling uneasy about hearing "footsteps behind me at night" in the neighborhood. The method of scale construction and the scale reliability are found in Greenberg, Rohe, and Williams (1984b, Appendix A).

[3]An attempt was made to use rates of personal, property, and nonindex crimes, but the high degree of multicollinearity among these variables ($r \geqslant .68$) precluded their simultaneous inclusion in the same equation.

by oblique rotation.[4] Based on the pattern of factor loadings, the three principal factors that emerged were interpreted to represent, respectively, housing deterioration (high loadings on trash and litter, building flaws, abandoned buildings, and vacant lots), single-family areas with little commercial land use, and single-family areas with few flats. The presence of rehabilitated housing was included in the regression analysis as a separate variable because of its low correlation with the other physical characteristics.

The variable identified as "All Problems" was a ten-item index of perceived neighborhood problems. These items reflect many of the dimensions of disorder and loss of control that are subsumed in the concept of incivilities. Indicators of local networks and perceived economic viability have been discussed previously. A term was added to express the interaction effect on fear of property appreciation and the perceived helpfulness of neighbors. Finally, an index was created to express an individual's social and physical vulnerability. Race and income are indicators of exposure to crime that results from social status, since the crime rate is typically higher in low-income, nonwhite areas. Sex and age are indicators of physical vulnerability. The index is the sum of standard (z) scores on each of the four variables; higher index values indicate greater vulnerability (i.e., being older, female, and nonwhite and having an annual family income below $10,000).

The results of the analysis appear in Tables 3.1 and 3.2. Standardized slopes (beta weights) are presented for the full model, as well as adjusted R^2s and change in adjusted R^2s contributed by the predictor variables at each step.[5] It might be argued that standard regression is inappropriate for one of the dependent variables, safety satisfaction, because it is dichotomous. For this reason, standard regression results with this dependent variable were checked against results obtained with discriminant analysis, a multivariate technique that is designed to be used with categorical dependent variables. No differences were found in the direction or relative strength of the partial relationships between the independent and dependent variables.[6] Standard regression was used

---

[4]For details of factor analysis and scale construction, see Greenberg, Rohe, and Williams (1984b; Tables A3-A5).

[5]The adjustment in R^2 refers to the correction made for the number of predictor variables relative to the number of cases.

[6]As a general rule, nonlinear multivariate statistical techniques will achieve the same results as standard linear regression as long as the distribution of the dichotomous dependent variable falls between 25% and 75% (Cohen & Cohen, 1975). In the case of safety satisfaction, 73% stated they were somewhat or very satisfied with the safety of their neighborhood, which falls just within the acceptable range.

TABLE 3.1. Regression of Safety Satisfaction on Crime, Physical Characteristics, Perceived Local Problems, Local Social Networks, Investment Satisfaction, and Vulnerability

Independent variable	Step entered into equation	Standardized beta	Adjusted R^2	Adjusted R^2 change
Total crime	1	−.001		
Victimization	1	−.153**		
Housing deterioration	1	−.028		
Single-Family/noncommercial	1	−.137**		
Single-Family/no flats	1	.022		
Rehabilitation	1	.038	.101**	.101
All problems	2	−.239**		
Low crime	2	.160**	.220**	.119
Helpful neighbors	3	−.050		
Know strangers	3	−.000		
Real home	3	−.030		
Community association	3	−.003	.217**	−.003
Good investment	4	.155**		
Housing quality	4	.146**		
Property appreciation/ Helpful neighbors interaction	4	.062	.260**	.043
Physical/social vulnerability	5	−.098*	.267**	.007

Note. Sources are the combined neighborhood survey and Housing and Neighborhood Appearance Rating survey, Taub, Taylor, and Dunham (1984).
*$p < .01$, **$p < .001$.

TABLE 3.2. Regression of Worry on Crime, Physical Characteristics, Perceived Local Problems, Local Social Networks, Investment Satisfaction, and Vulnerability

Independent variable	Step entered into equation	Standardized beta	Adjusted R^2	Adjusted R^2 change
Total crime	1	.018		
Victimization	1	.059		
Housing deterioration	1	.064		
Single-Family/noncommercial	1	.015		
Single-Family/no flats	1	−.063		
Rehabilitation	1	−.067	.103**	.103
All problems	2	.199**		
Low crime	2	−.172**	.186**	.083
Helpful neighbors	3	−.004		
Know strangers	3	−.010		
Real home	3	−.018		
Community association	3	−.010	.185**	−.001
Good investment	4	−.107*		
Housing quality	4	.012		
Property appreciation/ Helpful neighbors interaction	4	−.048	.193**	.008
Physical/social vulnerability	5	.226**	.237**	.044

Note. Sources are the combined neighborhood survey and Housing and Neighborhood Appearance Rating survey, Taub, Taylor, and Dunham (1984).
*$p < .01$, **$p < .001$.

here because of the more widespread familiarity with the statistics this method produces.

Safety Satisfaction

The regression of safety satisfaction in Table 3.1 shows that the perception of neighborhood problems related to order maintenance was the most important predictor of safety satisfaction; satisfaction decreased as the number of perceived problems increased. Other important predictors, all roughly equal in size, were perception of low neighborhood crime, satisfaction with housing quality and the neighborhood as an investment, residence on a single-family noncommercial block, and victimization. Of somewhat less importance was individual vulnerability. Perception of low crime and economic viability increased safety satisfaction, while victimization, vulnerability, and residence in a single-family area decreased satisfaction. The finding of a negative effect on satisfaction of residence on a block dominated by single-family dwellings is counterintuitive, and the explanation is not readily apparent. However, the other measures of physical deterioration had no direct effect on the dependent variable, nor did the reported crime rate. In addition, the indicators of local social networks had no significant effects on satisfaction.

The combination of perceived neighborhood problems and perceived crime level accounted for the largest percentage of explained variance, and increased the adjusted R^2 from .101 to .220. More than one quarter of the total variation in safety satisfaction was explained by the predictor variables.

Worry

Table 3.2 shows the regression results for the worry index. Individual vulnerability was the most important predictor of worry, followed closely by perceived problems and perception of low neighborhood crime. Perception that the neighborhood is a good investment is the remaining significant predictor of worry. None of the objective crime-related or physical characteristics was significant, nor were the social network variables. Of the significant predictors, the combination of perceived problems and low crime explained the highest percentage of the variation. The linear combination of all predictors accounted for almost one quarter of the variation.

The results thus far indicate that the findings for both indicators of fear are similar. The only exception is that household victimization is a significant predictor of safety satisfaction, but not of worry. It is, however, less important than perceived problems. In general, the most important predictor variables are perceived order-related problems, perceived crime level, satisfaction with health of the local housing market, and individual vulnerability.

On the other hand, physical deterioration and the local crime rate do not have direct effects on fear. Although these variables may be too far removed from the experience of fear to exert a direct influence, they may have an indirect effect through neighborhood perceptions. Indicators of local networks also were relatively unimportant. Perceived helpfulness of neighbors and sense that the neighborhood was a real home have a moderate negative relationship with fear on the zero-order level, but this may be a function of perceived problems and perceived crime; when the joint effect of one or both of these variables on social networks and fear is controlled, the relationship between networks and fear disappears. The effect of perceived economic viability remains, however, even after crime and order-related perceptions are controlled. This suggests that confidence in the economic well-being of the neighborhood is a buffer against fear in spite of the fact that an individual may be aware of neighborhood problems.

These suggestions of direct and indirect effects of variables at both the area level and individual level indicate a need to examine the causal path between objective neighborhood characteristics, perceptions related to neighborhood crime and control, and fear.

Path Model of Neighborhood Characteristics, Crime and Control-Related Perceptions, and Fear

The following analysis examines the intermediate relationships between objective neighborhood characteristics and fear, that is, the predictors of and the relationships among the crime and control-related perceptions that are hypothesized to transmit the effects of physical characteristics to fear. This analysis follows the causal logic that was illustrated in Figure 3.1. The dependent variables include (1) perceived control-related problems, (2) perceived level of neighborhood crime, (3) perceived helpfulness of neighbors, (4) ease of stranger recognition, (5) sense that the neighborhood is a real home, (6) membership in a neighborhood association concerned with the quality of community life, (7) perception that the neighborhood is a good investment, and (8) perceived housing quality. According to the model, dependent variables (1) and (2) are predicted by the objective crime rate, indicators of physical deterioration, and rate of property appreciation, as well as household victimization and individual vulnerability. The remaining dependent variables are predicted by the above independent variables plus perceived problems and

TABLE 3.3. Regression of All Problems on Crime, Physical Characteristics, and Vulnerability

Independent variable	Standardized beta	Adjusted R^2
Total crime	.092*	
Victimization	.227***	
Housing deterioration	.265***	
Single-Family/noncommercial	−.136***	
Single-Family/no flats	.061	
Rehabilitation	.006	
Property appreciation	.108**	
(1 = rapid, 2 = intermediate, 3 = slow)		
Physical/social vulnerability	−.011	.191***

Note. Sources are the combined neighborhood survey and Housing and Neighborhood Appearance Rating survey, Taub, Taylor, and Dunham (1984).
*$p < .05$, **$p < .01$, ***$p < .001$.

perceived crime level. Standard linear regression is the statistical technique utilized.[7]

Perceived Neighborhood Problems

The perception of control-related problems was regressed on crime, physical deterioration, and property appreciation (see Table 3.3). The most important predictors are housing deterioration and household victimization, followed by residence on a block dominated by single-family housing and little commercial land use, reported crime rate, and property appreciation. Although victimization appears to enhance the perception of problems, individual vulnerability does not. All relationships are in the expected direction, and almost one fifth of the variation in perceived problems is explained by the independent variables.

Implicit in the concept of disorder at the neighborhood level are crime and physical decay, as well as the breakdown of norms for public behavior. The findings indicate that, in fact, the perception of problems that are believed to reflect social disorder is predicted by a combination of crime and physical deterioration.

This is less true for perceptions of the level of neighborhood crime. In general, the independent variables explained much less (5%) of the

---

[7]As in the previous analysis, dichotomous dependent variables (low-crime, known strangers, real home, community association membership, good investment perceived housing quality) were also analyzed by the discriminant technique. There were no differences between regression and discriminant analysis in either sign or ranking of predictor variables. For those who are interested, simple correlations among the variables used in this analysis appear in Appendix B in Greenberg, Rohe, and Williams (1984b).

variability in perception of neighborhood crime than in perceived problems (data not shown). Tract-level reported crime was not statistically significant. But housing deterioration and victimization both increased the perception of neighborhood crime, and the presence of rehabilitated housing slightly decreased the perception of crime. These findings suggest that crime at the tract level may be too far removed to have an effect on individual crime perceptions.

Social Networks

Residence on a block dominated by single-family dwellings has positive effects on all four indicators of social networks (perceived helpfulness of neighbors, ease of stranger recognition, perception that the neighborhood is a real home, and membership in a local association concerned with the quality of community life). Tables 3.4 and 3.5 present the results for perceived helpfulness and ease of stranger recognition. In both cases, single-family residence has a significant positive effect. In fact, for perceived helpfulness, as for perception that the neighborhood is a real home and community association membership (data not shown), single-family residence is the single most important predictor variable. These results suggest that in residential areas with either mixed land use or a substantial proportion of multiple-unit dwellings, commitment and interaction are less likely to develop.

Other neighborhood characteristics had less consistent effects. Higher area crime rates dampened the perception of the neighborhood as a real home, while residents of areas with a slow rate of property appreciation were more likely to recognize strangers. This is probably a result of the

TABLE 3.4. Regression of Helpful Neighbors on Crime, Physical Characteristics, Vulnerability, and Perceived Local Problems

Independent variable	Step entered into equation	Standardized beta	Adjusted R^2	Adjusted R^2 change
Total crime	1	−.058		
Victimization	1	−.045		
Housing deterioration	1	−.057		
Single-Family/noncommercial	1	.215*		
Single-Family/no flats	1	.020		
Rehabilitation	1	.036		
Property appreciation	1	−.004		
Physical/social vulnerability	1	−.009	.112*	.112
All problems	2	−.175*		
Low crime	2	.062	.144*	.032

Note. Sources are the combined neighborhood survey and Housing and Neighborhood Appearance Rating survey, Taub, Taylor, and Dunham (1984).
*$p < .001$.

TABLE 3.5. Regression of Known Strangers on Crime, Physical Characteristics, Vulnerability, and Perceived Local Problems

Independent variable	Step entered into equation	Standardized beta	Adjusted R^2	Adjusted R^2 change
Total crime	1	−.061		
Victimization	1	−.046		
Housing deterioration	1	−.008		
Single-Family/noncommercial	1	.148***		
Single-Family/no flats	1	.037		
Rehabilitation	1	−.003		
Property appreciation	1	.208***		
Physical/social vulnerability	1	.105**	.114***	.114
All problems	2	−.012		
Low crime	2	.082*	.119***	.005

Note. Sources are the combined neighborhood survey and Housing and Neighborhood Appearance Rating survey, Taub, Taylor, and Dunham (1984).
*$p < .05$, **$p < .01$, ***$p < .001$.

greater stability of these neighborhoods, compared to neighborhoods with a higher demand for housing.

Individual characteristics also had less consistent effects. In general, victimization did not reduce local social contacts, and in fact, increased the likelihood of membership in a community association. The index of vulnerability had a positive effect on stranger recognition and perception of the neighborhood as a real home. Examination of the simple correlations suggests that this is primarily a function of the age component of vulnerability. Older people were more likely to recognize strangers and feel that the neighborhood is a real home, probably because they are less residentially mobile than are younger people. Blacks were less likely to feel that the neighborhood was a real home than were whites.

With regard to neighborhood perceptions, the greater the number of perceived problems, the lower the perceived helpfulness of neighbors and the less the sense of the neighborhood as a real home. Perceived problems did not encourage or discourage community association membership. Perception of low crime was positively associated with stranger recognition, although the causal path could go in either direction. Crime perception did not significantly affect the other indicators of local social networks.

The combination of the neighborhood, individual, and perceptual characteristics explained a moderate (for individual-level data) proportion of the variation in the dependent variables, 12% to 14%, with the exception of community association membership where only 3% was explained.

Perceived Economic Viability

The last two dependent variables are both indicators of perceived economic viability of the neighborhood—sense that the neighborhood is a good investment and satisfaction with the quality of housing for the money. In both cases, perceived problems was the single most important predictor; the greater the number of order-related problems, the less the confidence in the area's economic well-being (Tables 3.6 and 3.7). It should be noted that neither the crime rate nor the perceived crime level

TABLE 3.6. Regression of Perceived Housing Quality on Crime, Physical Characteristics, Vulnerability, and Perceived Local Problems

Independent variable	Step entered into equation	Standardized beta	Adjusted R^2	Adjusted R^2 change
Total crime	1	−.078		
Victimization	1	.005		
Housing deterioration	1	−.037		
Single-Family/noncommercial	1	.147*		
Single-Family/no flats	1	.014		
Rehabilitation	1	−.062		
Property appreciation	1	.013		
Physical/social vulnerability	1	−.133*	.122*	.122
All problems	2	−.280*		
Low crime	2	.031	.188*	.066

Note. Sources are the combined neighborhood survey and Housing and Neighborhood Appearance Rating survey, Taub, Taylor, and Dunham (1984).
*$p < .001$.

TABLE 3.7. Regression of Good Investment on Crime, Physical Characteristics, Vulnerability, and Perceived Local Problems

Independent variable	Step entered into equation	Standardized beta	Adjusted R^2	Adjusted R^2 change
Total crime	1	−.060		
Victimization	1	−.048		
Housing deterioration	1	−.085		
Single-Family/noncommercial	1	.103*		
Single-Family/no flats	1	.007		
Rehabilitation	1	.012		
Property/appreciation	1	−.164**		
Physical/social vulnerability	1	−.016	.100**	.100
All problems	2	−.202**		
Low crime	2	−.008	.130**	.030

Note. Sources are the combined neighborhood survey and Housing and Neighborhood Appearance Rating survey, Taub, Taylor, and Dunham (1984).
*$p < .05$, **$p < .001$.

had this effect. Residence on a block dominated by single-family housing and little commercial land use enhanced perceived economic viability. As would be expected, residence in an area undergoing rapid property appreciation enhanced the satisfaction with the neighborhood as an investment. It did not have this effect on perceived housing quality, since prices may increase dramatically in an area in which the housing is in need of extensive repair. Vulnerablity reduced satisfaction with housing, due primarily to the negative effects of being black or low-income. In general, confidence in the economic viability of the neighborhood was highest among people who perceived fewer order-related problems and who lived on blocks with primarily single-family housing and homogeneous land use.

Summary and Conclusions

Figure 3.2 summarizes the results of the analysis tracing the causal paths from objective neighborhood and individual characteristics, through the intervening perceptions concerning neighborhood crime, disorder, social networks, and economic viability, to the indicators of fear.

The analysis indicates that perceptions of disorder and crime and confidence in the economic well-being of the neighborhood were pivotal variables linking objective neighborhood characteristics with fear. Neighborhood crime did not have a direct effect on fear. Its effects were indirect via its effects on perceived order-related problems.

Perhaps the most important neighborhood characteristic was the proportion of single-family housing. It had a direct (though positive) effect on one measure of fear, as well as indirect negative effects on both fear measures through perceived problems and economic confidence. The effect of housing deterioration on fear was indirect through its effects on perceptions of problems and crime level.

Perceptions of crime and order-related problems both had strong direct effects on fear. Perceived problems also had an indirect effect as a result of its effect on economic confidence. Confidence in neighborhood economic viability had a negative effect on the indicators of fear.

Although the indicators of local social networks had a negative relationship with fear, as indicated by the simple correlations, when perceptions concerning local crime and other problems were controlled, these relationships became negligible. This suggests that perceptions of the helpfulness of neighbors and the neighborhood as a real home as well as fear are in part joint outcomes of crime and control-related perceptions; they do not appear to be causally related. Finally, victimization had a direct effect on fear as well an indirect effect through perceptions of local crime and problems.

Independent Variables	Dependent Variables											
	Perceived Problems	Perceived Low Crime	Helpful Neighbors	Know Strangers	Real Home	Association Member	Good Investment	Housing Satisfaction	Safety Satisfaction	Worry
Crime Rate	+				−					
Victimization	+	−							−	
Housing Deterioration	+	−								
Single-Family Block	−		+	+	+	+	+	+	−	
Rehabilitated Housing		+		+	+					
Property Appreciation	+			+			−			
Individual Vulnerability				+	+			−	−	+
Perceived Problems			−		−		−	−	−	+
Perceived Low Crime				+				+	+	−
Helpful Neighbors										
Know Strangers										
Real Home										
Association Membership										
Good Investment								+	+	−
Satisfaction– Housing Quality								+	+	

FIGURE 3.2. Summary of results of analysis of neighborhood crime, physical deterioration, neighborhood perceptions, and fear. Only those direct effects that are statistically significant at $p < .05$ are reported.

The results suggest that enhancing confidence in the economic well-being of the neighborhood and reducing perceptions of both local crime and problems related to order maintenance will have the effect of reducing fear. The evidence also indicates that these perceptions are most strongly affected by the level of housing deterioration, residence in a single-family area, and victimization experience. However, local social networks did not have a direct effect on fear. In general, the area crime rate did not influence perceptions related to neighborhood conditions, even crime-related perceptions.

In summary, these findings indicate that if fear of crime does, in fact, help to destroy social life in contemporary urban communities, strategies aimed at fear reduction primarly through fostering contacts among neighbors may be less than optimal. The evidence points to the importance of strengthening the economic well-being and sense of confidence in neighborhoods as well as reducing victimization in the effort to reduce fear.

Acknowledgments: This is a revised version of a paper presented at the meeting of the American Society of Criminology, Denver, Colorado, November 1983. The research from which this paper was developed was supported under the auspices of Grant No. 81-IJ-CX-0080 from the National Instutite of Justice, Community Crime Prevention Division. The study was completed while the author was at the Research Triangle Institute and the Denver Research Institute. This paper benefitted from input by William Rohe, University of North Carolina-Chapel Hill.

4
Delinquency Rates as Sources of Ecological Change

ROBERT J. BURSIK, JR.

Introduction

Ecological studies of local community rates of crime and delinquency have formed one of the important ongoing traditions of empirical criminology. One of the most significant theoretical advances in the interpretation of such spatial distributions was made by Shaw and McKay (1931, 1942) when they argued that neighborhood differentials in delinquency rates could only be fully understood when considered within the context of broader urban dynamics. However, as Kornhauser (1978, pg 118) has noted, they never explicitly formulated the causal linkages that connected such processes of urban growth with delinquency but only emphasized the *mutuality* of the interrelationships. Likewise, most of the ecological research that has followed in the tradition of Shaw and McKay (such as Bordua, 1958-59; Chilton, 1964; Chilton & Dussich, 1974; Gordon, 1967, Lander, 1954) has concentrated primarily on estimating the levels of association between crime and/or delinqucy rates and various sociodemographic indicators of community composition without evaluating a specific causal framework.

Nevertheless, this body of research has generally assumed (either implicity or explicity) that the level of delinquency in a community is dependent on these sociodemographic compositional elements. More general human ecologists, however, have stressed that the elements of the "ecological complex" (see, for example, Duncan & Schnore, 1959) are reciprocally related. In fact, Duncan and Schnore (1959, p. 139) have noted that it is this dual process of adaptation that "some writers have identified as the most fundamental premise in ecological thinking" and Berry and Kasarda (1977, P.15) argue that it gives the ecological approach its heuristic value in the study of change. Organization, of course, is one of the central components of the ecological complex. Therefore, if local delinquency rates are important indicators of community organization, as suggested by Shaw and McKay (1942), there may not be a simple, unidirectional causal structure in which crime and delinquency rates are only the outcome of ecological processes. Rather, within the context of ongoing urban dynamics, the level of delinquency in an area may also directly or indirectly cause changes in the composition of an area.

The dynamics underlying mutual causal effects at the local community level have been suggested by the recent neighborhood research of Taub, Taylor, and Dunham (1981, p.118) who argue that high crime rates may become symbolic of perceived neighborhood deterioration. Although it has often been assumed that such perceptions make out-migration from an area more likely, Katzman (1980) has noted that the overall relationship is not especially strong. However, he did find that upper middle-class families were significantly more likely to move out of such neighborhoods, thus changing the relative composition of the area. In addition, he also found that certain groups (such as families with higher incomes and/or children) were especially sensitive to issues of crime when making neighborhood destination choices; this implies that crime rates may have an effect on the types of people who move into certain local communities.

Thus, if movement into or out of a neighborhood becomes significantly more likely for certain sociodemographic goups under these conditions, then crime rates have themselves accelerated or altered the ongoing processes of comunity change. A related argument has been presented by Watts and Watts (1981) in their discussion of the relationship between crime rates and the percentage of blacks in large cities. Many studies have found a strong positive relationship between these variables and have concluded that "blacks have 'reasons' to commit crimes" (Watts & Watts, 1981, p. 425).[1] However, Watts and Watts argue that the interpretation of this relationship is far from clear since the direction of causality has not been determined; rather, they suggest that the process of suburbanization may have left minorities "stranded in high crime areas" (p.424). Their nonrecursive model of crime rates during 1970, in fact, supports just such a conclusion: although the percentage of non-whites does not significantly affect the crime rate in large cities, the crime rate does have a strong positive effect on that percentage.

The finding of Watts and Watts (1981) cannot be directly generalized to local community processes for two reasons. First, cities rather than neighborhoods are the unit of analysis, and the related ecological processes are more centrally associated with issues of the impact of a city's facilities and economic activities on the remainder of the local geo-

---

[1]Typical interpretations noted by Watts and Watts (1981;pp. 425-426) include "a positive cost/benefit, frustration, lack of allegiance to a social contract or the system, lack of absorption into society or, perhaps, a culture of poverty."

graphic area (see Gibbs & Erickson, 1976; Stafford & Gibbs, 1980, p.653) than the processes of invasion and succession which are considered the central ecological dynamics within cities.[2] In addition, given the restriction to only 1970 crime rates, it is not possible to determine the extent to which such conclusions would be modified if lagged relationships were also included in the model. Nevertheless, their important finding indicates that the uncritical acceptance of a unidirectional ecological process resulting in local rates of delinquency may be highly misleading.

Data and Initial Model Specification

The delinquency data analyzed in this paper were collected under the direction of Henry McKay while he was at the Institute for Juvenile Research in Chicago and reflect the rates (per 1,000 male juveniles) of male delinquency referrals to the Cook County, Illinois, Juvenile Court during 1960 and 1970 for each of the local community areas of Chicago.[3,4] The social composition of the local areas is reflected in seven socio-demographic indicators drawn from census materials and aggregated to the local community level: the percentage of nonwhites (NW), the percentage of foreign-born whites (FB), the percentage of the male labor

---

[2]It should also be noted that problems of the "ecological fallacy" may also arise in such a generalization, for one would be trying to infer processes found in one type of aggregation from those found in another.

[3]An unfortunate aspect of the delinquency data is that we cannot determine the nature of the offense for which the youth was referred. Given the nature of court-derived official data, it is fairly safe to assume that the rates reflect the incidence of relatively serious types of delinquency. However, we recognize that there may be offense-specific differences in the processes discussed in this paper that we regretfully cannot discuss.

[4]As of 1980 there were 77 such areas; however, only 75 were recognized to exist in 1960; in addition, we have eliminated one community area from the analysis (#32—the Loop) due to its very small juvenile population, resulting in an N of 74 communities.

A very detailed description of the origin of these areas can be found in Kitagawa and Taeuber (1963; see also Hunter, 1974). They were originally delineated in the 1930s to reflect the Chicago schools' notion of natural areas and do not entirely coincide with neighborhoods that are currently recognized to exist, although there is a great deal of overlap. Kitagawa and Taeuber have defended their use in the following way: "There has been a deliberate attempt to maintain a constant set of subareas within the city in order to analyze changes in the social, economic and residential structure of the city...redefining boundaries every ten years would destroy the usefulness of the grid for studying change" (p.xiii).

force that is unemployed (UNEMP), the percentage of professional, technical, and kindred workers (PROF), the percentage of owner-occupied dwellings (OWNOCC), the percentage of households with more than one person per room (DEN), and the median education level (ED). The choice of indicators was guided by two considerations. Due to the nature of the larger project from which this report is drawn, the measures had to be consistently available from 1940 through 1970. In addition, they had to reflect the racial, housing, and economic dimensions discussed in other ecological works of this kind.

Those readers familiar with our past work may wonder why the entire dataset (1940-1970) has not been used to estimate the model. As Heise (1975) and Kenny (1979) have argued, causal analysis is only appropriate when the structure underlying a system of variables is not undergoing change during the period of analysis. This is definitely not the case in Chicago during this 30-year period. Through a confirmatory factor analysis of the delinquency rates and sociodemographic indicators for 1940, 1950, 1960 and 1970, Bursik (1984) has shown that an important change in the associational structure was apparent during 1950 that was related to changes in black residential patterns resulting from the open-housing decisions of 1948. In addition, the ecological structure of Chicago's neighborhoods became significantly more complex after 1940, confirming Hunter's (1974) observation concerning Chicago's ongoing differentiation. However, there was evidence of at least a temporary stabilization in this process during 1960 and 1970: a test of the equality of the correlation matrices for these years could not reject the null hypothesis. Therefore, it was decided that a great deal of simplification in the initial analysis of the mutual causation hypothesis was possible if the model was first fit in terms of this stable structure. A full understanding of such ecological dynamics, of course, will only be possible when such models can account for temporal variations in these structures. This consideration will form an important part of our future work.

In building and evaluating ecological models of delinquency, severe problems of multicollinearity arise since most of the sociodemographic indicators that are considered reflect concurrent outcomes of ongoing processes of residential invasion and succession (Bursik & Webb, 1982). This is a primary reason why factor analysis has been one of the major approaches to such data. Yet, although such approaches minimize the problems of multicollinearity when incorporated into regression models (Chilton & Dussich, 1974), it is not clear how many factors are needed to adequately describe the ecological structure. The maximum likelihood procedure used in the analysis of Bursik (1984) needed four factors to fit the correlation matrices of 1960 and 1970. However, as Gorsuch (1974) has illustrated, this is no guarantee that four is the "correct" number of factors: Monte Carlo simulations have indicated that maximum likeli-hood approaches derive an *upper* bound to the underlying dimensionality of a correlation matrix. On the other hand, Gordon (1967) has emphasized the use of the 1.0 eigenvalue criterion for determining the number of factors. This approach is also not faultless, for as Gorsuch (1974) again points out, this has been shown to provide a *lower* bound for the number of dimensions. In addition, the eigenvalue criterion is a mathematical rather than statistical approach in that the sampling variance of the factor structure cannot be determined. For example, while the eigenvalue criterion indicated that two factors should be kept for the 1960 solution and *three* for the 1970 solution, recall that the test of equality provided no evidence of a significant difference between these 2 years, implying that the underlying factor structures are also equivalent.

For the purposes of this research, we have restricted the dimensionality of the sociodemographic indicators to that produced by a principal, two-factor solution. As will be seen, the two-factor model leads to the derivation of underlying dimensions that are easily interpretable and we feel that in such an essentially exploratory approach to the issues discussed previously, it is preferable to work from simple models and build to the complex. In addition, however, such a restriction has the added benefit of making the solution substantively very similar to the two-factor solutions for Baltimore, Detroit, and Indianapolis presented by Gordon (1967),[5] leading to a greater generalizability of the findings.

The sociodemographic factors incorporated into the analysis are presented in Table 4.1. The first dimension (RACE) represents a combination of the racial composition, unemployment rates, and housing status found in Chicago's communities. However, the RACE label is used primarily for convenience, since the factor has a very strong economic aspect to it. Gordon(1967) has argued that the ecological correlation between socioeconomic status and delinquency rates is predominantly a function of the lower end of the economic distribution. Given the especially strong loadings for unemployment rates and household density, we argue that this dimension reflects the prevalence of this end of the economic continuum in a community, which also differentiated between the living situations of whites and nonwhites during this period of Chicago's history. The second dimension (SES), therefore, can be interpreted as reflecting the degree to which the upper end of this continuum is present in a neighborhood.

A full examination of the role of delinquency rates in the ecological process must consider two important potential effects. First, certain neighborhoods may have established reputations as high crime areas and

---

[5]We must emphasize that although similar structures appear in these cities, it is premature to assume that they reflect stable, ongoing ecological patterns associated with delinquency . See the argument of Bursik (1984).

TABLE 4.1. Ecological Constructs of the Causal Model (Factor Loadings)

Indicators	1960		1970	
	RACE	SES	RACE	SES
NW	.961	−.187	.925	.041
FB	−.764	−.047	−.632	−.108
UNEMP	.888	−.417	.866	−.255
PROF	−.281	.686	−.283	.619
OWNOCC	−.468	.357	−.480	.015
DEN	.823	−.452	.852	−.398
ED	−.029	.754	.099	.711

are not considered to be attractive locations of residence. In such a situation, delinquency may be expected to have a lagged effect on the composition of an area in that past levels affect current patterns of residence. In addition, there may also be "instantaneous" effects in the sense that rapid increases in rates of delinquency may lead to a relatively simultaneous compositional change due to the concerns of residents about the future of an area.

Unfortunately, the dual analysis of lagged and instantaneous effects presents two technical problems of statistical identification for the model. When the ecological structure is viewed as a system of relationships, such as is the case here, the number of measured correlations must be greater than or equal to the number of causal parameters to be estimated. This is not the case when both types of effects are considered (see the discussion of cross-lagged panel correlations by Kessler & Greenberg, 1981); therefore, a predetermined set of restrictions had to be made. We decided to regress each construct in 1970 on the corresponding construct in 1960 and utilize the residuals as the 1970 indicators.[6] This approach eliminates three of the paths from the system since the correlation between the 1970 residuals and the 1960 predictors is necessarily 0. However, the benefits of such an approach are far more than statistical. As Kessler and Greenberg have noted (1981, P.8), correlations between time 1 and time 2 measurements of the same variable confound the degree of stability and predictable change in that variable. Since we are most centrally interested in the extent to which delinquency rates can modify other ecological processes, the use of the residual as the time 2 variable has the important

---

[6]The resulting residuals are usually called "residual change scores." The R^2 values resulting from the regression of the 1970 constructs on the 1960 measurements were .64 for RACE, .56 for DEL, and .44 for SES.

theoretical advantage of representing changes in the levels of the ecological constructs that are not expected on the basis of their initial levels. In addition, since all of the communities are used to estimate the regression equations upon which the residuals are computed, the change scores automatically reflect a community's position vis-á-vis the general dynamics characterizing the city as a whole. This is especially pertinent given Shaw and McKay's (1929;1942) argument concerning the role of broader urban dynamics in giving meaning to local community processes.

Therefore, for example, a significant negative lagged relationship between DEL60 and SES70 would imply that the level of delinquency in a neighborhood was related to *subsequent* unexpected decreases in that area's socioeconomic status that are not attributable to the prior status of that community. Relatedly, a significant negative relationship between DEL70 and SES70 (both of which are residual change scores) would denote that unexpected increases in the delinquency rate may have fairly *immediate* effects on changes in the economic composition of an area.

The hypothesized ecological process based on the presumed existence of both of these effects and the use of the residual change scores is presented in Figure 4.1, which illustrates the second identification problem of the model. In general, at least as many exogenous variables (the 1960 constructs) must be eliminated from an equation as endogenous variables (the 1970 constructs) are included for the instantaneous effects to be identified. Therefore, the equation for RACE70 (=f(DEL70, DEL60, SES60)) is just identified since only one endogenous variable is included and one exogenous variable is excluded. However, the equation for DEL70 (=f(RACE70, SES70, RACE60, SES60)) is underidentified since there are two endogenous variables included in the equation but only one exogenous variable excluded. In order to make these effects over-identified (so that statistical tests become meaningful), we have added three instrumental exogenous variables into the analysis, each related

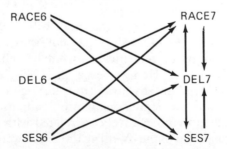

FIGURE 4.1. Hypothesized model. All 1970 constructs are residual change scores computed on the basis of the corresponding 1960 constructs. The effects of the three instrumental variables are not shown.

fairly strongly to one of the endogenous variables and only weakly to the others: the percentage of the population receiving public aid in 1970 (as an instrument for RACE70), the suicide rate in 1970 (DEL70), and the percentage employed in blue collar occupations (SES70). It should be emphasized that these instruments were for substantive as well as empirical reasons. The role of the public aid indicator, for example, is motivated by our previous argument that the RACE factor actually reflects both the ethnic/racial composition of an area and the degree to which that area is characterized by the lower end of the economic distribution; the small correlation between public aid and SES70 (.055) supports this assumption. Similarly, the suicide rate has been incorporated as an instrument for DEL70 on the basis of Shaw and McKay's argument (1929,1942) that such rates are also a reflection of the degree of social disorganization in a community. Although these instuments have been used to estimate the model, their effects will not be discussed in the following sections since they are secondary to the primary focus of this paper. However, interested readers can regenerate these parameters on the basis of Table 4.2, which presents the intercorrelations among all of the variables in the analysis. The model was estimated through a two-stage least-squares approach.

Findings

Gordon's (1967) discussion of the Baltimore, Detroit, and Indianapolis data reported a very weak relationship between median rent and delinquency rates; similar findings have been reported by Polk (1957-58) in San Diego for measures of occupation and education. Therefore, the finding that SES has neither a lagged nor concurrent effect on DEL (Figure 4.2) is not especially surprising. However, the finding that high rates of delinquency are strongly related to subsequent significant increases in SES is completely unexpected and, on first consideration, very counterintuitive.

Although a full understanding of this path will necessitate some very subtle future analysis, the relationship may not be as surprising as it first seems given the process of gentrification that has characterized many U.S. cities since the 1970s. Henig's research (1980) suggests that these young professionals tend to "shy away from hard-core inner city tracts"; increases in the relative compositon of professionals in the neighbor-hoods that he studied were negatively correlated with the percentage of blacks and the proportion of the dwelling units that were renter-occupied. Such findings are entirely consistent with the negative path from RACE60 and SES70. Although comparable evidence concerning the role

TABLE 4.2. Matrix of Intercorrelations

	RACE70	DEL70	SES70	RACE60	DEL60	SES60	Public aid	Suicide	Blue collar
RACE70	1.000								
DEL70	0.478	1.000							
SES70	0.281	0.125	1.000						
RACE60	-.000	0.003	0.026	1.000					
DEL60	0.238	0.000	0.245	0.692	1.000				
SES60	-.364	-.079	-.000	-.101	-.398	1.000			
Public Aid*	0.340	0.149	0.055	0.837	0.800	-.452	1.000		
Suicide*	-.104	-.238	-.079	-.288	-.193	-.114	-.241	1.000	
BLCOLLAR*	0.206	0.090	-.445	-.109	0.058	-.619	0.095	0.073	1.000
Means	-0.000	0.000	0.000	0.000	15.568	0.000	7.478	0.085	34.649
S.D.	0.599	7.220	0.632	1.006	12.120	0.871	8.950	0.062	9.365

*Instrumental variables

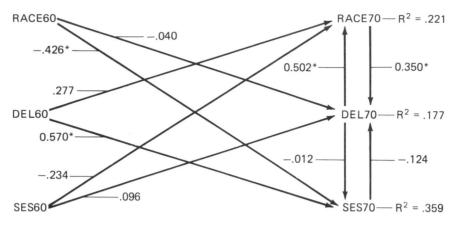

FIGURE 4.2. Two-stage least squares estimates of parameters. All coefficients are standardized; effects which are more than twice their standard error are marked with an asterisk. Although R^2 values are note totally reliable in nonrecursive models, they have been included for informational purposes.

of delinquency rates in the gentrification process is not available, the possiblity that potential "gentrifiers" may be attracted to non-minority neighborhoods characterized by single-family-dwelling- units in areas of high delinquency is plausible since the costs of housing may be less than in other low-crime, nonminority areas. It should also be noted that this positive correlation does not appear to be related to the effect of outliers in the data[7] and that a similar "perplexing" pattern has been reported in at least one other city. In their recent longitudinal analysis of Los Angeles, Schuerman and Kobrin (1983) report that although there is a negative relationship between socioeconomic status in 1950 and the crime rate in 1960, the relationship is moderately positive between 1960 and 1970. Although their evidence is based on a reversal of the path that is discussed here, it does indicate that the relationship beteen SES and DEL has undergone some important recent changes in large urban areas that are deserving of further consideration. Whatever the correct explanation may be, however, it is apparent that delinquency rates have an important effect on the nature of other ecological processes.

On the other hand, the relationship between the items included in the RACE construct and delinquency has been recognized for a long time and, as Watts and Watts (1981) note, it is generally assumed that RACE

---

[7]The use of Cook's D as a test for influential observations did not indicate that any of the communities had an undue effect on the form of the functional relationship between DEL6 and SES7.

has causal priority. Such a conclusion must be strongly modified in light of Figure 4.2. First, while the racial composition of an area does not appear to be related to subsequent increases in deliquency, unexpected increases in RACE do appear to cause simultaneous increases in DEL. Bursik and Webb (1982) have interpreted such a relationship in terms of neighborhood organization and the finding is consistent with several existing ecological theories of crime as well as the original formulation of Shaw and McKay (1929,1942). What such theories do not predict, however, is changes in the delinquency rate also cause unexpected changes in the RACE factor and, more importantly, the standardized magnitude of this path is almost 1½ times the size of the traditionally considered relationship. Most likely, this confirms Watts and Watts' (1981) proposal that in such situations those who are able to leave the neighborhood do so, resulting in an increase in the relative proportion of minority and very poor residents in the area. Such a proposition cannot be resolved definitively without data on residential mobility. Nevertheless, it is again apparent that delinquency rates in themselves play an important role as agents of ecological change.

Conclusions

Despite the great volume of literature on ecological processes and delinquency, there is still a fairly rudimentary understanding of the role played by crime in the overall dynamics of urban development. Although the research reported here represents a modest attempt to refine our understanding of these processes, two general findings appear to have very important implications for theory development. First, delinquency rates are not simply the outcome of ecological processes in large urban areas. Rather, at least in Chicago, they are important components of that process and have been shown to have an important effect on the dynamics of urban change in that they can greatly accelerate ongoing patterns of neighborhood transition. This finding is especially crucial in that it calls into question generally accepted interpretations of the race-crime association at the neighborhood level. Although changes in racial composition cause increases in the delinquency rate, this effect is not nearly as great as the effect that increases in the delinquency rate have on minority groups being stranded in a community. The theoretical implications of the possible gentrification effect are not clear, for this may repesent a temporary ecological aberration. However, if the gentrification phenomenon continues, an area's delinquency rates (in conjunction with their effect on housing values in nonminority areas) may significantly affect future patterns of settlement and redevelopment.

Second, and more generally, the analysis stresses the importance of grounding our ecological theories of crime and delinquency more fully in broader studies of urban change. Schuerman and Kobrin (1983), for example, can only give meaning to the patterns found in Los Angeles after a consideration of the long-term dynamics of urban development and neighborhood change. Bursik and Webb (1982) were forced to consider the macrosocial effect of new laws concerning open housing that in turn changed the residential settlement patterns of minority populations in order to resolve an apparent contradiction of Shaw and McKay's approach (1929,1942). Likewise, in this paper, the relationship between DEL60 and SES70 would have been incomprehensive without a consideration of recent patterns of inner-city resettlement.

Although a general theory of urban change was central to the work of Shaw and McKay (1929,1942), the discipline seems to have drifted away from such an integration of perspectives in recent years. Many very important urban phenomena described by noncriminological sociologists which have significant implications for the study of crime (such as the role of the defended community) have yet to appear in ecological theories of crime. Yet, until such considerations are made, our understanding of the ecology of crime and delinquency will continue to be, at best, rudimentary.

Acknowledgments: This is a revised version of a paper presented at the 1983 annual meeting of the American Society of Criminology, Denver, Colorado. The author would like to thank Parker Frisbie, Harold Grasmick, James Lynch, Don Merten, Charles Tittle, and Jim Webb for their review and comments. This research was funded in part by Grant #84-IJ-CX-0071 awarded by the National Institute of Justice.

Part II Interurban Analyses of Violent and Property Crime

5
Cities, Citizens, and Crime: The Ecological/Nonecological Debate Reconsidered

JAMES M. BYRNE

Introduction and Overview

Over the past 50 years, a great deal of thought, not to mention a considerable body of empirical research, has been directed at a deceptively simple question: Why do some cities have higher rates of crime and other forms of "unconventionality" (e.g., conflict, suicide) than others? Not surprisingly, most researchers have begun their examination of intercity variation in crime rates by looking at the gross variation in index crime rates by city size. What we invariably find is "a monotonic relationship between crime rates and the size of the reporting jurisdiction" (Chaiken & Chaiken, 1983, P.17). In 1980, for example, the index crime rate in very large cities (i.e., cities with populations over 250,000) was almost *twice* as high as the comparable small city (i.e., cities in the 10,000-25,000 population range) rate (9,356 vs. 5,346 per 100,000 pop.).[1] How can we explain these differences? Is there something (inherently bad) about the *structure* of larger cities or the *individuals* who reside in them which could explain these findings? Or does the answer lie elsewhere?

In the following analysis, four related questions about intercity variation in crime rates will be addressed: (1) Do the physical characteristics of communities have an independent effect on the level of different types of property crime, once population compositional characteristics are controlled? (2) How much improvement does a general model of intercity variation in property crime (i.e., robbery, burglary, larceny, motor-vehicle theft), which includes both physical and population-compositional variables, represent over existing "models" of property crime? (3) Do these models change dramatically when we examine larger

---

[1] See Jan M. Chaiken and Marcia R. Chaiken, "Crime Rates and the Active Criminal," p. 17, Table 2, in James Q. Wilson (1983).

and smaller (i.e., cities over vs. cities under 100,000 population) cities separately? (4) Does the nature of the interaction between physical characteristics and population-compositional variables change when we examine different types of property crime (e.g., robbery, burglary)? Answers to these questions should improve our understanding of the relation between "city life" and crime. It is in this context that we will be able to assess the competing claims of ecological and nonecological theorists.

The Ecological/Nonecological Debate

The relationship between cities and crime can be described from both an ecological and a nonecological perspective. The ecological theorists (as exemplified by Louis Wirth, 1938, 1964), hypothesize that the physical characteristics of cities (e.g., size, density, division of labor) have a significant and strong effect on both property and violent crime.[2] Michael Smith (1979), in his exegesis of Wirth's theoretical perspective, provides a succinct synopsis of Wirth's view of the link between size, cultural disorganization, and crime:

... The multiplicity of conflicting subcultures found in the urban mosaic impedes the development of common cultural understandings that might regulate behavior informally. This absence was viewed by Wirth as a basic cause of crime and delinquency. (P.21)

In direct contrast, the nonecological or compositional theorists (as exemplified by Herbert Gans, 1962) deny the central importance of physical characteristics or "ecological" variables.[3] To Gans and other "compositionists," the Wirthian perspective ignores the fact that:

... social integration—and consequently, psychological well-being too—is sustained within small, private, social worlds even in the largest cities... Thus, urban residence does not, according to the critics, cause interpersonal estrangement, nor its subsequent effects. (Fischer, 1981, p. 307)

Compositional (or nonecological) theorists believe that it is the characteristics of city residents (class, social mobility, age composition, ethnicity, etc.) that "explain" intercity variation in crime rates. More specifically, physical characteristics are hypothesized to have no significant effect on the crime rate once relevant population-compositional characteristics are controlled.

Who is correct? A review of the existing research suggests neither.

---

[2]In particular, see Louis Wirth, "Urbanism as a Way of Life," in Albert J. Reiss, Jr. (1964). See also, Wirth (1938).
[3]See Herbert Gans (1968).

According to Fischer (1975), it is the *non*ecological position that is most commonly accepted in the field of sociology, despite the fact that individual traits simply do not account for the differences between "belief and behavior" (including, of course, crime) in urban and rural areas.[4] When viewed separately, both the (traditional) ecological perspective and compositional theory offer incomplete explanations of the city-crime correlation reported at the outset of this paper. Thus, it appears that an integrated theoretical perspective is needed which takes into account the nature of the *interaction* between personal characteristics of population aggregates and the physical characteristics of cities.[5]

Testing an Integrated Ecological Model

The examination of person-environment interactions is consistent with a view of human ecology as the study of the relation of persons to, and the interaction of persons with, the environment.[6] The concept of ecological complex (Duncan & Schnore, 1959) provides a convenient analytical and theoretical framework for studying these interactions. According to Hauser and Schnore (1965):

The "ecological complex". . . has four basic components: environment, population, social organization and technology. These variables are seen as functionally interrelated: a change in one leads to modifications in the others. (p. 165)

I will adapt this approach (i.e., the ecological complex) in the following analysis.[7] By utilizing this conceptual framework it is possible to view the city from an interactionist perspective.[8]

---

[4]See Fischer (1975). Fischer emphasized that, while there is little empirical evidence to confirm Wirth's urban alienation hypothesis, "the association between urban residence and unconventionality is pervasive" (p. 1322).

[5]Gottfredson and Taylor (chapter 8, this volume) take a similar approach (using neighborhood) in their study of parolees in Baltimore. In particular, see their discussion of the Olweus' person-environment integrity model. Of course, the interactionist perspective is exemplified by Lewin (1936).

[6]Clearly, this is *not* what most criminologists would describe as the ecological approach. Most of us still link ecology and crime to work of the Chicago School of Social Ecology which included Burgess, Park, and Shaw and McKay, or perhaps more specifically, the zonal model of cities and crime. However, after reviewing these early efforts (and the subsequent critiques) Bottoms concluded that "ecology in the full sense as delineated by Park is justly discredited" (Baldwin & Bottoms, 1976, p.14).

[7]For a critique of this approach, see Gideon Sjoberg, "Theory and Research in Urban Sociology," Chapter 5, in Hauser and Schnore (1965).

[8]A more detailed discussion of the ecological complex is found in Chapter 2 in Byrne (1983).

Ideally, a study based on this perspective would include characteristics of population aggregates (e.g., race, income, family composition) along with characteristics of the physical environment (e.g., density, overcrowding, opportunity, size of place). The former group of variables focus on characteristics of a city's aggregate *population* and also on its social *organization*; the latter groups of variables identify elements of the physical *environment* and describe the role of *technology* (e.g., weight of household items, availability of victim stock).[9]

However, in the present study, general ecological models of property crimes which highlight *two* key elements (i.e., population and environment) of the ecological complex have been constructed and validated. A more complex approximation of the ecological complex of Duncan and Schnore was not possible.[10] Nonetheless, by including both the social characteristics of population aggregates (e.g., ethnicity, poverty) and essential elements of the physical environment (e.g., size, density) in the following analysis, I offer a preliminary test of the competing claims of ecological and nonecological theorists regarding the nature of the relation between cities and crime.

Specifically, both physical and population-compositional characteristics have been employed to develop structural models of *property crime* in a sample of over 900 cities in the United States. My decision to focus exclusively on property crime was based primarily on the fact that few empirical investigations of property crime in the United States have ever been conducted and as a result, a number of questions concerning the etiology, patterns, and control of crimes for gain have gone unanswered.[11]

---

[9]Cohen (1981) recently suggested that criminal opportunities are affected by more general technological changes. For example, the increased number of lightweight goods (e.g., TV sets, stereos) available to steal has, in essence, made burglary easier and more profitable.

[10]Because two elements of the ecological complex—technology and social organization—were measured inadequately, any statements about the applicability of a general ecological model are equivocal, underscoring the preliminary nature of the analysis.

[11]I will analyze four types of "crime for gain" in this study: robbery, burglary, larceny, and motor vehicle theft. Although there is some debate over whether robbery should be classified as a violent or a property crime, I conclude that since the "outcome" of the crime is, essentially, acquistion of property, it can be viewed as a property crime. However, in the case of robbery (and, in fact, all property crimes), this may not be the only *motive*. Nonetheless, as Sparks, Greer, and Manning (1982) observed:
... what (at most) can be said about theft, fraud, etc. is that a *typical immediate motive* for doing such things is the acquisition of something that is useful, beneficial, valuable, etc, to the perpetrator; and the "something" seems in most cases to be of at least a minimally tangible kind. Money is of course the paradigm; things that can be turned into money also qualify. (p. 59)

Some Basic Propositions About the Social Ecology of Crime

An earlier review of the available research on cities and crime by the author (Byrne, 1983) suggested that we will find crime-specific, size-specific, and region-specific variation in the ecological (and noneco-logical) correlates of property crime in American cities.[12] Nonetheless, the general ecological model tested in this study is based on the following assumption: *Both* the physical and population-compositional character-istics of cities help explain variation in the rates of specific types of property crime. Necessarily, then, both sets of variables are expected to have an independent effect on the crime rate, and this independent effect should remain even if (1) larger and smaller cities are analyzed separately, and (2) regional analysis is conducted.

The need for a size-specific analysis was underscored by Harries (1980), who pointed out that there may be variation in the correlates of city crime rates which is obscured when we group together geographic units which are not homogeneous. Treating city size as a predictor variable does not directly address this issue, since an *overall* property crime rate (i.e., for all cities) is still used, rather than a size-specific criterion. By developing ecological models of each type of property crime based on a simple size categorization, we can examine possible variation in the magnitude of the correlations as well as in the relative importance of physical and population-compositional characteristics across cities in different size categories. This strategy—dividing the sample into specific size categories and rerunning the regression analysis—is suggested in research conducted by Flango and Sherbenou (1976). They found that the magnitude of the correlations between their independent and dependent variables were stronger in the larger (i.e., cities over 100,000) than in the moderately sized cities.[13]

Furthermore, even among cities of the same general size category, homogeneity should not be assumed; there may be variation within these two subgroups and by region of the country. For example, it is an empirical question whether a city of 25,000 in an otherwise under-populated western state is comparable to a city of the same size which is in the eastern part of the country and surrounded by a number of larger cities. This also touches on the need to consider the ecological position (i.e., SMSA/city population ratio and dominance [city/SMSA retail

---

[12]See Chapter 2 in Byrne (1983). Harries (1980) has reported similar variations in violent and property crime.

[13]These findings may not be accurate, however. Briefly, the authors' initial factor analysis included *all* cities; but, at one point, they used the extracted factors as independent variables in separate regression analyses of large and small cities. They should have redone their factor analysis for each subsample of cities (i.e., those over and under 100,000). The same problem biased their finding of regional variation in crime correlates.

sales]) of each city in the sample (Stafford & Gibbs, 1980). While the data needed to include ecological position are not available for all cities in the sample, we can, at the very least, examine the homogeneity issue among those cities for which data are available. Moreover, regional variation in *robbery* models may be explained in terms of variation in the ecological position of cities in different parts of the country.[14] Once again, Flango and Sherbenou (1976) took a similar approach in their analysis of the differential impact of poverty in southern states.

Research Procedures

The present study can be discussed in terms of three distinct stages: (Phase 1) the initial bivariate analysis (data cleaning and reduction) stage: (Phase 2) the construction stage; and (Phase 3) the validation stage. First, three random subsamples of cities have been drawn from the total sample of 910 cities included in the Country and City Data File. About 10% (n = 95) of the sample is included in Phase 1; by comparison, 460 cities are in the Phase 2 subsample. The remaining 355 are found in Phase 3. The distribution of cities across the three subsamples reflects my belief that: (1) a small initial sample of cities is adequate for the initial data cleaning, reduction, and analytical procedures; and (2) a somewhat larger construction sample should reduce the shrinkage of the estimated crime models (Simon, 1971).[15]

In Phase 1 the initial bivariate analyses were conducted. It is here that

---

[14]According to Gibbs and Erickson (1976), this variable can only be measured for the (approximately) 400 cities in my study with populations over 50,00. They observed that:

... 50,000 was taken as the minimum limit because cities of that size are necesarily parts of a Standard Metropolitan Statistical Area (SMSA) and an Urban Area (UA) (though they may not be central cities). Unless a city is part of a SMSA and a UA, one cannot compute an approximation of the community/city size ratio [and the city/SMSA retail sales measure]. (p.612)

However, it appears that there are also cities between 25,000 and 49,999 in population for which the corresponding SMSA totals can be obtained. Why? Unlike these authors, I am not interested in *only* cities in both UAs and SMSAs; some cities in this size range are outside UAs but within SMSAs.

[15]It is interesting to note that the 5 boroughs of New York City were inadvertantly included as separate cities (*along with N.Y.C.*) in the County and City Data Book. The boroughs were removed from this study. For a discussion of the issue see Byrne (1983: Chapter 4). The comparability of the three randomly selected subsamples can be directly assessed by examining Appendix A, Table 1, in Byrne (1983).

the issues of multicollinearity, nonlinearity, and outlier cities were resolved.[16] The main purpose of Phase 2 was to estimate the parameters of the initial (12) crime and size-specific regression models to be validated in Phase 3. For each of the four property crimes examined (robbery, burglary, larceny, and motor-vehicle theft), three equations were estimated: an all-city model (n = 356); a bigger-city model (n = 75); and a smaller-city model (n = 281). Similarities and differences between the bigger-city and smaller-city models were examined at this point, and the relative importance of physical and population-compositional variables was assessed. Four regional models of robbery (Northeast, North Central, South, and West), were also developed and compared.[17]

In the final phase of the analytical design (Phase 3), each of the models of property crime estimated in Phase 2 was validated on a separate, random sample of 351 cities.

Data Sources

The unit of analysis employed in this study is the *city*.[18] The primary data source is the 1977 County and City Data File, which includes a wide variety of census data describing 910 cities in the United States with a 1975 population of at least 25,000. (Only 18.6% of the cities of this file [i.e., larger cities] have 1975 population totals over 100,000; We refer to the remaining cities as "smaller.") The data file has two primary advantages: (1) it provides a more refined unit of analysis than has been used in almost every macroenvironmental study of cities and crime; (2) it

---

[16]For a fuller discussion of these issues, see Chapter 4 Byrne (1983).

[17]See Kowalski et al. (1980) for a discussion of regional crime patterns. In addition, see Flango and Sherbenou's (1976) analysis of the culture of poverty in Southern cities.

[18]The selection of the city as the "appropriate unit" of analysis in a macro-environmental study of crime is not discussed here. (See Byrne, 1983, for a discussion of this issue.) However, a note on the "definition" of cities is in order. Walton and Carns (1973) have observed that:

The concept "city" has not always meant what it does today, and probably will not mean the same thing in the future. As we use the term now, a city consists of a relatively dense population living off an agricultural hinterland, with or without manufacturing, but with some form of interdependence and specialization of functions. (p.11)

Briefly, use of such concepts as Gibbs and Erickson's (1976) "ecological position" allows us to explore this interdependence without using the entire SMSA as the unit of analysis. For a somewhat different perspective, see Hoch (1974) or Stafford and Gibbs (1980).

includes the largest number of cities that is currently available for a study of the ecological correlates of crime.[19] Despite some limitations, the data are available to offer a preliminary test of the general ecological models of each property crime presented here.

Predictor Variables

To examine the competing claims of ecological and nonecological theorists, both *person* (i.e., population-compositional characteristics) and *environment* (i.e., physical context of cities) variables must be included in the analysis. Previous research on cities and crime has suggested that a large number of person and environment factors must be examined initially.

Population-compositional variables reflect the aggregate characteristics of the people who live in a particular area. Stahura, Huff, and Smith (1978) suggest a typology of population-compositional variables which includes ethnicity, income, and age composition. However, criminological research has also focused on the relation between a number of other population-compositional variables and crime, suggesting this basic typology should be expanded. The following population-compositional variables are included in the first phase of the analysis: ethnicity (percent white), age composition (percent 18-25 years of age), income (median family income), poverty (percent below poverty level), employment diversity (percent employed in manufacturing, wholesale and retail trade, and government), and a variety of other factors—that is, education (percent persons over 25 years of age who completed 4 or more years of high school), citizenship (percent foreign stock in a city), and gender (percent female). While the above listing is not exhaustive, it does include a multiplicity of aggregate characteristics of city residents which have been correlated with property (and violent) crime in previous intercity analyses.[20]

A number of variables reflecting characteristics and components of the physical environment in American cities are also included in this study. Previous intercity analyses suggest that the following physical charac-

---

[19]Only the number of cities used by Flango and Sherbenou (1976) is comparable (n = 840 cities).

[20]Other population compositional variables which should be included in subsequent analyses (at least in the initial phases) are population change, unemployment stability, residential mobility, family composition, and female labor-force participation rate. (For a complete review of these variables, see Chapter 4 in Byrne, 1983.)

teristics of cities are related to property (and violent) crime: density (population per square mile), overcrowding (percent with 1.01 or more persons per room), city size (total population), region (Northeast, North Central, South, and West), division of labor (mix of manufacturing, wholesale trade, retail trade, and service establishments in an area), commercial differentiation (mix of 15 specific retail and service establishments), and housing factors (median housing value, median gross rent, percent single-family units, percent owner-occupied units, and percent lacking some or all plumbing facilities). Once again, the above listing is not exhaustive, although the major characteristics of the physical structure of cities have been employed.[21]

In summary, both physical characteristics and population-compositional variables have been correlated with property (and violent) crime rates in a number of previous intercity analyses. Nonetheless, it should be emphasized that not only the *number* of variables employed but also the *measures* of these variables vary from study to study, making a simple summary of findings misleading.

Identifying the Criterion

Research on intercity variation in crime rates has focused on a range of criterion variables (See the review in Byrne, 1983.). If a general trend can be discerned, it is that we are moving in the direction of improved offense-refinement. Four types of criterion variables have been used: (1) overall crime rates; (2) rates of violent and property crime; (3) crime-specific rates (e.g., robbery, burglary); and recently, (4) rates based on intracrime categories (e.g., residential vs. bank robbery). Why does the choice of criterion matter? To answer simply, it matters because crime is not a unitary phenomena and factors which may be associated with the level of one type of crime (e.g., larceny) may not be associated with another type (e.g., burglary). If, for example, in an ecological study of crime, robbery, larceny, motor-vehicle theft, and burglary were included in a general property crime rate, we would not know whether the factors related to the overall property crime rate were also related to each crime category, unless we conducted a separate crime-specific analysis. Even then, however, there could be variation *within each crime category*. Would an ecological study of bank robbery identify the same macrovariables as

---

[21]Other physical characteristic variables which have been employed in previous studies include the employment/residence ratio, structural density, technology, community age, occupational diversity, climate, and seasonality. (For a complete review, see Chapter 4 in Byrne, 1983.)

a similar study of residential or commercial robbery? While this type of analysis has rarely been conducted, some recent findings by Shichor, Decker, and O'Brien (1979) concerning the relation between population density and crime directly address this issue. They identified variation within specific crime categories (robbery, larceny, burglary, and assault) in the relation between density and crime, and suggested that "much of the inconsistency in the findings concerning the relationship of population density and crime rates may be due to treating different types of crime as a unitary phenomenon" (Shichor, Decker & O'Brien, 1979, p. 186). This potential source of bias was present in every other study I reviewed (Byrne, 1983). It is also a problem in the present study. Individual property crime categories will be examined; possible intracategory variation, however, will not be explored.

Four types of property crime will be analyzed in this study: robbery, burglary, larceny, and motor-vehicle theft. Uniform Crime Report (UCR) definitions of each of these crimes will be used. The problems and limitations of this data source have already been noted elsewhere.[22] but one further caveat is in order: The level of underreporting of crime to the police varies by type and category. For example, victimization data reveal that, in 1976, slightly over one half of all personal robberies were reported to the police, while almost 9 out of 10 commercial robberies were reported. Thus, reported robbery totals misrepresent the actual mix of robbery types by underestimating personal robberies. Similarly, about one-half of all burglaries were reported, but commercial burglaries were reported more often than residential burglaries. In contrast, completed motor-vehicle thefts were only reported 91% of the time; however, "attempted" motor-vehicle thefts were only reported in 39% of all cases. The reporting of larceny thefts to the police varied by the amount of property lost: 14% of larceny under $50, but 54% of larceny over $50 was reported in 1975. Taken together, these data suggest that the extent of the "errors in variables" problem inherent in using offenses known to the police to measure crime is not "uniform," either across or within categories of crime (McCaghy, 1980). This is an important factor to remember when examining the differences in the ecological correlates of each property crime between larger and smaller cities; in a very real sense, we may be comparing apples to oranges.

---

[22]Sparks, Glenn, and Dodd (1977) commented on the continued study of *official* crime rates despite their incompleteness and inherent bias:

For most of the past century, the 'dark figure' of unrecorded crime has been rather like the weather: criminologists all talked about it, at least in the first chapters of their textbooks, but none of them; did very much about it. (p. 2)

In this respect, I am a lot like "most criminologists." My only defense is that the corresponding victimization data for these 910 cities is simply not available.

Findings

Phase 1: Bivariate Analyses

The results of the initial bivariate analysis are only briefly summarized here (for a more detailed presentation, see Byrne, 1983). Three potential problems are focused on which were identified and solved: multicollinearity, nonlinearity, and outliers. To begin, all large-scale ecological studies must be aware of potential *multicollinearity* problems since the preliminary list of predictors are often intercorrelated. Indeed, a quick perusal of the zero-order correlation matrix including all predictors (table not included) reveals that multicollinearity (i.e., conservatively, any correlation greater than .60) is present in 12 pairs of variables.[23]

Table 5.1 summarizes the variable-selection procedure by identifying the reason each variable was included in the analysis. Clearly, a number of variables were added for *theoretical* reasons which were unimportant at the bivariate level. It should also be noted that if one of the final list of

---

[23]Michael Lewis-Beck (1980) outlines the common solutions to this problem. See also Holmes (1979, 1981); Belsley, Kuh, and Welsh (1980); Farrar and Glauber (1967); and Rockwell (1975).

TABLE 5.1. Summary of Key Variables to be Employed in the Phase 2 Analysis[a]

	Robbery	Burglary	Larceny	Motor-vehicle theft
City size	.3704*	.3798*	.2197**	Added
Density	Added	Added	Added	Added
Overcrowding	Added	.1701*	Added	Added
Percent single-family	—	—	—	−.3381*
Percent owner-occupied	−.3345*	−.1769**	Added	—
Population ratio	Added	Added	−.2778*	Added
Dominance	Added	Added	.2603*	Added
Commercial differentiation	−.2499*	−.1730**	Added	−.2357*
Ethnicity	−.4393*	−.4813*	Added	Added
Percent youth	Added	Added	Added	Added
Average family income	Added	−.1684**	Added	—
Poverty	—	—	—	Added
Percent foreign-born	—	Added	Added	.3315*
Education	—	—	—	Added
Employment diversity	—	.1874**	—	—

Note.— = not included. Added = Added for theoretical reasons.
[a]Region will also be included in the Phase 2 analysis, using dummy variables.
*$p < .01$. **$p < .05$.

variables in Table 5.1 was not used, it was always because of the multicollinearity problem. This accounts for the crime-specific differences in the number and type of variables added for theoretical reasons.

A number of researchers have raised the issue of possible nonlinearity in many crime-ecological correlations (e.g., Beasley & Antunes, 1974; Mladenka & Hill, 1976). Examination of the scatterplots of the bivariate correlations between all predictor variables and each type of property crime revealed that nonlinearity was indeed a problem with each of the following variables: city size, density, overcrowding, percent white, median family income, percent foreign born, and poverty. For this reason, logged versions of these variables were used in multiple regression analysis.

The general pattern of outliers in the Phase 1 sample was also analyzed (no figures included; but see Byrne, 1983). Clearly, we can greatly improve the fit of the bivariate correlation if we simply delete the small number of outliers identified.[24] For this reason, the outliers identified in the next analytical stage will be dropped from the Phase 2 sample. Maximizing the explanatory power of the regression equation is viewed as the primary object of the first two analytical phases, and the elimination of outliers is a necessary step in this direction.

Overall, results of the Phase 1 bivariate analysis (no tables included) revealed that for each property crime, the magnitude, strength, and direction of these correlations vary by size of place. The simple dichotomization of city size produced some very startling differences in the size of bivariate correlations, underscoring the importance of place in this analysis.[25]

Phases 2 and 3: Model Construction and Validation

The results of the Phase 2 multiple regression analysis are presented in Tables 5.2 through 5.5. In addition, each property crime model was validated using a separate, random sample of 351 cities. I will begin with a discussion of the validation findings.

Briefly, the purpose of the validation procedure is to test the results of the multiple regression analyses (i.e., the parameter estimates for equations 1-12) on another unique data base. This process allows the

---

[24]Indeed, when the cities identified as outliers are dropped from the analysis, the corresponding correlations often change dramatically. See Chapter 4 in Byrne (1983).

[25]For example, marked differences in the *size* of the correlations can be identified for *robbery*. The bivariate correlation between percent youth (18-to 25-year-olds) and robbery is $-.47$ for the larger cities, but .04 for the smaller cities.

researcher the opportunity to assess the "goodness of fit" of his or her model, while at the same time estimating the extent to which overfitting the data occurred. The researcher can then present an unbiased estimate of the power of the parameters of the regression equation(s).

Inspection of Table 5.2 reveals that of the original 12 models, the robbery equations fit the best ($R^2 = .51-.67$) and the larceny equations fit the worst ($R^2 = .10-.15$). In addition, the motor-vehicle theft equations "shrunk" the most, suggesting some overfitting of the data during the (Phase 2) construction stage. Clearly, if the validation phase had been ignored, I would often have *over*estimated the importance of the variables included in my ecological models of each property crime. Perhaps more important, the degree of overestimation varied by the *type* of property crime studied.

With the validation results in hand, we can examine each of the initial

TABLE 5.2. Summary of Validation Results

Equation number	Description	Construction sample R^2	Validation sample R^2	Difference (c-v)[a]
1	Robbery—All cities	.67	.67	—
2	Robbery—Big cities	.57	.58	+.01
3	Robber—Small cities	.54	.51	−.03
4	Burglary—All cities	.36	.30	−.06
5	Burglary—Big cities	.20	.05	−.15
6	Burglary—Small cities	.34	.25	−.09
7	Larceny—All cities	.14	.10	−.04
8	Larceny—Big cities	.21	.15	−.06
9	Larceny—Small cities	.13	.10	−.03
10	Motor-vehicle theft—All cities	.42	.30	−.12
11	Motor-vehicle theft—Big cities	.38	.48	+.10
12	Motor-vehicle theft—Small cities	.27	.16	−.11
13	Robbery—Big cities with population dominance	.75	.64	−.11
14	Burlary—Big cities with population dominance	.26	.09	−.17
15	Larceny—Big cities with population dominance	.20	.30	+.10
16	Motor-vehicle theft—big cities with population dominance	.54	.38	−.16
17	Robbery—Northeast cities	.78	.78	—
18	Robbery—North Central cities	.73	.72	−.01
19	Robbery—Southern cities	.74	.63	−.11
20	Robbery—Western cities	.41	.38	−.03

Note: The construction sample R^2 represents the amount of variance explained by the simplified model used in the equations.
[a]Difference between R-square in construction and validation samples (Diff: c-v).

"hypotheses" about size and crime-specific variation in the ecological and nonecological correlates of property crime, since we now have unbiased estimates of the explanatory power of our crime, area, and region-specific models. To my knowledge, the present (cross-sectional) study is the first intercity analysis to utilize a validation sample in this manner.

At the outset of this paper some preliminary propositions were presented which are consistent with an integrated socio-ecological perspective on cities and crime and reflect my attempt to provide a preliminary test of the "ecological complex." My first hypothesis was that both the physical and population-compositional characteristics of cities would be associated with each of the four property crimes examined. The present research supports this contention.

Next, it was proposed that the relative importance of physical and population-compositional variables would vary by the *type of crime* being examined.[26] A comparison of the "all city" regression results supported this hypothesis. (Table 5.3 highlights this finding.) For robbery, a population-compositional variable (percent white: Beta = −.46) was the most important predictor, but physical characteristic variables accounted for 9 of 12 significant correlations. For burglary, another population-compositional variable, median family income (Beta = −.30), was the most important predictor; however, three of the four remaining significant correlates were physical characteristics.

In contrast, Northeast (a physical characteristic) had the highest correlation with larceny (Beta = −.32); only percent foreign born (a population-compositional variable) and percent owner-occupied were also significantly correlated with this property crime. Finally, another physical characteristic, percent single-family housing (Beta = −.31), was the largest correlate of motor-vehicle theft; six other variables (three physical and three compositional variables) were also significantly correlated with this crime type. Clearly, crime-specific variation in the relative importance of these two groups of variables has been identified.

My third hypothesis was that *both* physical and population-compositional variables would be significantly correlated with each type of property crime regardless of size of place. The results of the size-specific analysis are presented in Table 5.4. The robbery and burglary results supported this hypothesis; the larceny and motor-vehicle theft findings

---

[26]This hypothesis uses somewhat misleading terminology. "Relative importance" simply refers to the *size* of the standardized regression coefficient (Beta) for a particular variable in each of the four crime-specific all-city regression analyses. Here we are comparing the same sample of cases *using the construction sample* (n = 356).

TABLE 5.3. A Comparison of Ecological Correlates of Each Property Crime Standardized Regression Coefficients (Betas) (Construction Sample: n = 356)

Variables included in at least one equation	Property crime variables			
	Robbery	Burglary	Larceny	Motor-vehicle theft
Physical characteristics				
City size, log	.33	.22	.03*	.24
Density, log	.12	−.04*	−.04*	.04*
Overcrowding, log	−.02*	−.02*	.00*	.07*
Percent owner-occupied housing	−.14	−.18	−.17	—
Percent single-family housing	—	—	—	−.31
SMSA/City population ratio	.14	.11*	.00*	.10
Dominance (city/SMSA retail sales)	−.13	−.04*	.12*	−.18
Commercial differentiation	−.09	.02*	*	.01*
Northeast	−.10	−.06*	−.32*	.02*
South	−.13	.09*	.14*	−.04*
West	.01	.26	.11*	.02*
Population compositional variables				
Ethnicity (percent white)	−.46	−.21	−.04*	−.03*
Youth (percent 18–25)	−.11	−.07*	−.01*	−.12
Median family income, log	−.20	−.30	−.01*	—
Percent families below poverty, log	—	—	—	.15*
Percent foreign-born, log	—	.11*	.15	.12
Percent 25+ with 4 years education	—	—	—	−.17
**Construction R^2	.67	.36	.14	.42
**Validation R^2	.67	.30	.10	.30

Note.—= Not included.
*Not significant at .05 level.
**These are for the simplified models, using only significant ($p < .05$) correlates.

do not. Indeed, for both the larceny and motor-vehicle theft models, only *physical* characteristics are significantly correlated with the criterion in the separate big-city and small-city analyses. This finding does not support the notion presented at this study's outset concerning the need to integrate ecological and "nonecological" variables into a general ecological model of property crime. Such a general model would not be sensitive to the type of crime and area-specific variations described here.

A fourth hypothesis was that the significant correlates of each type of property crime will vary by the size of place; Moreover, there should also

TABLE 5.4. Results of Size-Specific Regression Analysis

Variables included in at least one equation	Robbery			Burglary
	All cities	Cities >100,000	Cities <100,000	All cities
Physical characteristics				
City size, log	.33	.31	.16	.22
	(86.2)	(100.9)	(67.1)	(233.4)
Density, log	.12		.12	
	(36.4)	(ns)	(30.2)	(ns)
Overcrowding, log	(ns)	(ns)	(ns)	(ns)
Percent owner-occupied housing	−.14		−.17	−.18
	(−2.0)	(ns)	(−.20)	(−10.5)
Percent single-family housing	—	—	—	—
SMSA/city population	.14		.19	
ratio	(0.5)	(ns)	(0.5)	(ns)
Dominance (city/SMSA	−.13	−.21		
retail sails)	(−102.5)	(−197.0)	(ns)	(ns)
Commercial differentiation	−.09		−.13	
	(−20.3)	(ns)	(−27.5)	(ns)
Northeast	−.10		−.12	
	(−51.7)	(ns)	(−51.0)	(ns)
South	−.13		−.13	
	(−67.7)	(ns)	(−55.6)	(ns)
West	.01			.26
	(2.8)	(ns)	(ns)	(512.0)
Population composition variables				
Ethnicity (percent White)	−.46	−.36	−.48	−.21
	(−579.7)	(−454.2)	(−565.)	(−1058.1)
Youth (percent 18–25)	−.11	−.23	−.12	
	(−2.8)	(−10.5)	(−2.4)	(ns)
Median family income,	−.20		−.22	−.30
log	(−193.1)	(ns)	(−163.5)	(−1183.8)
Percent families below				
poverty, log	—	—	—	—
Percent foreign born, log	—	—	—	(ns)
Percent 25+ w/4 yrs education	—	—	—	—
All numbers rounded to nearest whole number				
Construction R^2	.67	.57	.53	.36
Validation R^2	.67	.58	.51	.30

Note. These are the standardized (beta) and unstandardized (b) coefficients from the construction sample regression analyses. To examine the relative importance of a single variable *across* equations, you should examine the unstandardized (b) coefficients and standard errors. ns = F not significant at .05 level. — = not included.

Burglary		Larceny			Motor vehicle theft		
Cities >100,000	Cities <100,000	All cities	Cities >100,000	Cities <100,000	All cities	Cities >100,000	Cities <100,000
(ns)	(ns)	(ns)	(ns)	(ns)	.24 (123.8)	(ns)	.23 (212.0)
(ns)	(ns)	(ns)	(ns)	(ns)	(ns)	(ns)	(ns)
(ns)	(ns)	(ns)	(ns)	(ns)	(ns)	(ns)	(ns)
(ns)	-.25 (-14.4)	-.17 (-16.9)	(ns)	-.21 (-21.0)	—	—	—
—	—	—	—	—	-.31 (-6.8)	-.42 (-10.1)	-.32 (-6.8)
-.49 (-34.3)	.13 (1.7)	(ns)	-.55 (-64.0)	(ns)	.10 (0.7)	(ns)	.18 (0.9)
(ns)	(ns)	(ns)	(ns)	(ns)	-.18 (-270.1)	(ns)	-.20 (-305.3)
(ns)	(ns)	(ns)	.29 (322.2)	(ns)	(ns)	(ns)	(ns)
(ns)	(ns)	-.32 (-1134.1)	-.54 (-1932.2)	-.30 (-1013.2)	(ns)	(ns)	(ns)
(ns)	(ns)	(ns)	(ns)	(ns)	(ns)	(ns)	(ns)
.43 (887.6)	.25 (453.7)	(ns)	(ns)	(ns)	(ns)	(ns)	(ns)
(ns)	-.25 (-1384.1)	(ns)	(ns)	(ns)	(ns)	(ns)	(ns)
(ns)	(ns)	(ns)	(ns)	(ns)	-.12 (-5.9)	(ns)	(ns)
(ns)	-.22 (-794.6)	(ns)	(ns)	(ns)	—	—	—
—	—	—	—	—	(ns)	(ns)	(ns)
.40 (385.9)	(ns)	.15 (260.2)	(ns)	(ns)	.12 (59.2)	(ns)	(ns)
—	—	—	—	—	-.17 (-5.2)	(ns)	(ns)
.20	.34	.14	.21	.13	.42	.38	.27
.05	.25	.10	.15	.10	.30	.48	.16

be variation in the strength of these correlations when the big-city and small-city models are examined separately.[27] This hypothesis was supported for each property crime.

One final hypothesis was explored: that the ecological correlates of robbery will vary from one region of the country to another. The current research supports this contention. As you can see in Table 5.5, there are very high correlations between ecological variables and robbery in Northeastern and North Central cities ($R^2 > .70$), and Southern cities ($R^2 = .63$); There is only a moderate correlation between ecological variables and robbery in Western cities ($R^2 = .38$). In addition, there is regional variation in the ecological context of robbery: This is highlighted by the fact that (1) only population-compositional characteristics are significantly correlated with robbery in North Central cities, and (2) that the type of variables included in each regional model (and the strength of the correlations) also varies.

We now need to reassess the competing claims of ecological and nonecological theorists in light of these findings.

Conclusions

The results of this intercity analysis revealed that the importance of characteristics of the physical environment and the (aggregate) characteristics of the people who live in these environments varied by type of crime, size of place, and, for robbery, region of the country. Overall, neither the ecological nor the nonecological perspective alone offers an adequate explanation for these findings.

Larceny

To begin, it was found that the general ecological model of larceny tested in this study explained very little of the total intercity variation in larceny rates (i.e., for all cities at validation, only 10% of the variance explained). One justification for our inability to explain larceny is that the type of opportunity for larceny will vary *within* this crime type, making the use of an overall larceny-theft rate misleading. Simply stated, we need a more refined criterion which distinguishes shoplifting, pocket-picking, purse-snatching, thefts from motor vehicles, and other forms of larceny-theft. For example, it may be that the factors affecting shoplifting (e.g., surveillance) are quite distinct from the correlates of purse-snatching

---

[27]No specific tests were conducted to establish the significance of these differences. This approach has been criticized by some. See, for example, Chapter 2 in Rich, Sutton, Clear, and Saks (1982.)

TABLE 5.5. Comparison of Regional Models of Robbery (Unstandardized Coefficients: Construction Sample)

	Northeast (b)	North Central (b)	South (b)	West (b)	All cities[a] (b)
City size, log	93.322	35.810	82.719	89.118	86.248
	(24.55)[b]	(22.75)	(19.65)	(23.46)	(11.87)
Density, log	58.527*	24.981*	81.408	9.872*	36.404
	(36.08)	(22.19)	(23.89)	(23.46)	(12.92)
Overcrowding, log	60.430*	45.074*	-90.811	4.76*	-6.669*
	(54.53)	(29.99)	(36.90)	(28.77)	(17.07)
Percent owner-occupied units	2.471*	-2.355*	-.944*	-2.644*	-1.997
	(1.55)	(1.34)	(1.52)	(1.36)	(0.68)
Population ratio	-.772*	-.319*	.438*	.975	0.495
	(.51)	(.28)	(.876)	(.28)	(0.15)
Dominant	-33.470*	-72.544*	-64.647*	-147.250	-102.528
	(92.51)	(62.87)	(57.66)	(69.99)	(34.61)
Pop domi	49.328	3.835*	4.286*	58.942	(not used)
	(24.36)	(3.24)	(27.61)	(27.06)	
Com diff	-13.613*	7.981*	-20.623*	-49.127	-20.342
	(26.47)	(12.99)	(12.19)	(16.51)	(8.07)
Percent White	-1057.935	-1065.658	-449.521	-274.373*	-579.721
	(117.55)	(111.70)	(70.97)	(157.54)	(50.45)
Youth 1	-7.868*	-4.158	-2.043*	-2.645*	-2.80
	(4.69)	(1.51)	(1.59)	(1.72)	(0.97)
Medium Family Income, log	-130.221*	-75.969	-110.441*	-374.291	-193.094
	(120.89)	(126.13)	(92.05)	(116.82)	(57.90)
R^2	.83	.78	.77	.60	.80
Simplified R^2	.78	.73	.74	.41	.68
(Constant)	(4,552.964)	(5,216.321)	(2,053.256)	(4,263.796)	(3,674.37)
n	(71)	(115)	(78)	(92)	(356)

[a]Unstandardized coefficients for regions were also included in this model: Northeast (b = -51.689); South (b = -67.671); West (b = 2.802) were all significant (p < .05).
[b]Standard errors are in parenthesis.
*Variable not significant at .05 level.

(e.g., density). These differences are obscured when we use an overall larceny rate.

Motor-Vehicle Theft

The results of the motor-vehicle theft analyses underscored the need for a size-specific analysis. When all cities were included in the analysis, both physical characteristics (such as city size, percent single-family housing, population ratio, and dominance) and population-compositional variables (such as percent youth 18-25 years old, percent foreign born, and percent over 25 years of age with at least a high-school education) combined to explain a moderate amount (R^2 = .30 at validation) of the intercity variation in motor-vehicle theft rates. This supports my contention that intercity variation in property crime rates can only be explained by examining person-environment interactions. However, when the bigger and smaller cities were examined separately, we found that only characteristics of the physical environment (in particular, percent single-family housing) were significantly correlated with motor-vehicle theft. More importantly, these "ecological" models explained much more variation in larger cities than in smaller cities (R^2 = .48 and .16 at validation respectively). The implications of these findings for the ecological/nonecological debate are straightforward: the nonecological perspective does not hold up very well. It appears that cities (especially larger cities) with a higher than average proportion of single family housing have lower motor-vehicle theft rates, perhaps because of the existence of various buffering, protective devices, such as garages and the less anonymous single-family-dominated residential neighborhoods.[28] Of course, as we found with larceny, we do a poor job of explaining intercity variation in the motor-vehicle theft rates of smaller cities.

Burglary

A very different pattern emerged from the burglary analyses. When separate big- and small-city analyses were conducted, it was apparent that *better* relationships were achieved between both sets of variables in smaller rather than larger cities (validation R^2 = .25 and .05, respectively). This finding is surprising, and apparently contradicts the research of Flango and Sherbenou (1976). It appears that different ecological variables are affecting burglary rates in larger and smaller cities.[29]

---

[28]See Sampson (1983) for a discussion of this issue.

[29]For example, there are striking differences in the impact of the SMSA/city population ratio on burglary in larger versus smaller cities. The unstandardized coefficient (b) is −34.2 for cities over 100,000 but b = 1.7 for cities under 100,000. (See the discussion in Byrne, 1983, pp. 366-368.)

While we had little success explaining intercity variation among larger cities, we had a moderate degree of success in smaller cities. For the smaller cities, burglary rates were somewhat higher (1) in cities in the West, (2) in cities with a higher percentage of blacks, (3) in cities with a relatively smaller percentage of owner-occupied units, and (4) in cities with lower medium family incomes. Thus, an "integrated" burglary model (based on the ecological complex of Duncan & Schnore, 1959) is needed, but only for smaller cities. It is unclear which factors will explain intercity variation in burglary among larger cities.

Robbery

Finally, the present study has contributed most to our understanding of intercity differences in robbery rates. It appears that a combination of physical characteristics and population-compositional variables affect the robbery rate of U.S. cities. This suggests that both the ecological and nonecological perspectives offer incomplete explanations of intercity variations in robbery rates, and that attempts at integrating (and reconciling) these perspectives (e.g., Fischer's subcultural theory of urbanism) should continue. Stronger relationships were found between these ecological variables and robbery than for the other three property crimes. This points to the importance of ecological factors in an explanation of intercity variations in robbery rates. In particular, both ethnicity (race) and city size (place) are central to any explanation of intercity differences in robbery rates. The race or place dichotomy (Laub, 1980) is a crucial aspect of the ecological/nonecological debate. To many, the correlation between minority concentration (size) and a city's robbery rate represents the quintessential manifestation of the "blaming the victim" syndrome (e.g., see Blau & Blau's (1982) discussion of relative deprivation) which pervades social policy in the criminal justice arena today; to others, these findings suggest the need to examine the social relationships and values of our minority population (e.g., see the discussion of the subcultural perspective by Rosenfeld, Chapter 7, this volume). For this reason these two factors have been highlighted below.

City Size and Robbery
City size (logged) was significantly correlated with the robbery rate in all cities in the construction sample (Beta = .33). Not unexpectedly, the larger cities in the sample had higher robbery rates. This relationship persisted when bigger cities (Beta = .31; b = 100.9) and smaller cities (Beta = .16; b = 67.1) were analyzed separately. However, the comparatively smaller unstandardized coefficient for the cities with populations under 100,000 is worthy of some speculation.

If we assume Claude Fischer's (1975) notion of urbanization (i.e., that as city size increases the degree of urbanization increases), we find some persuasive evidence that the nonecological position (e.g., Gans, 1962; Lewis, 1965) greatly underestimates the importance of this factor in an explanation of intercity variation in robbery rates. In Fischer's view:

[The nonecological] position ... asserts there are few differences between urban and rural populations; those which do exist are attributable to differences in age, ethnicity, life cycle or social class—*not to any autonomous effect of ecological factors* [italics added]. (1975, p. 321)

Clearly, the nonecological position is not buttressed by the persistence of the city size-robbery correlation. In fact, the finding that city size was more central to an explanation of robbery rates in larger than smaller cities suggests that Fischer's idea of "critical mass" may be operating in cities with populations of about 100,000 or more. Once this critical mass (i.e., city size) is reached, subcultural size (within cities) is at a level where subcultural self-support, perpetuation, and intensification is possible. As size increases beyond this "critical mass" point, higher rates of unconventionality are observed.

One final note on the size-robbery correlation seems pertinent: When regional trends in the ecological correlates of robbery were examined, city size was again significantly correlated with the rate of robbery in Northeast cities (Beta = .30), Southern cities (Beta = .39), and Western cities (Beta = .36); However, size was not significantly associated with robbery in North Central cities (Beta = .13; $p > .05$). This final correlation suggests support for the nonecological position in this region only, a finding which is, at best, perplexing.[30]

A number of other researchers (Flango & Sherbenou, 1976; Harries, 1976; Hoch, 1974; Webb, 1972) have also found a (moderate to strong) positive correlation between city size and both violent and property crime. One project in particular deserves special attention. Flango and Sherbenou followed a strategy similar to the one taken in the present study. They divided their sample (n = 840) into two parts (i.e., cities over and under 100,000) and then assessed the relative importance of "socioeconomic environmental factors" in explaining crime in larger versus smaller cities. The authors pointed out that smaller cities have rarely been examined because researchers simply assumed that the same factors that explained high crime rates in larger cities would explain low crime rates in smaller cities. They concluded that this was decidedly not the case, since:

... *better* relationships were achieved between our six hypothesized criminogenic factors and crime in larger rather than in moderate-sized cities, especially with regards to the crimes of robbery [and motor-vehicle theft]. (Flango & Sherbenou, 1976, p. 343)

---

[30]Clearly, we have no reason to expect such regional variation from the nonecological perspective. But perhaps the distribution of larger and smaller cities in the North Central region affected the size-robbery correlation.

Both these authors and I have reached similar conclusions about the differential impact of urbanization[31] (or size) on the robbery rate in larger versus smaller cities: *It is a more important factor in larger cities.* The confluence of these findings (1) highlights the inherent bias of large city studies of robbery, and (2) underscores the need to analyze homogeneous subgroups of cities. A simple dichotomization of city size represents one step in this direction; yet it is a strategy very few researchers have employed.

Ethnicity and Robbery

Ethnicity (i.e., percent white) had the single largest correlation with the robbery rate when all cities in the construction sample were examined. Clearly, cities with the highest concentration of whites[32] had the lowest robbery rates. (Stated in its typical form, percent black was strongly correlated with high robbery rates.) Recent macroenvironmental research by Harries (1976, 1980), Quinney (1966), Schuessler (1962), Stafford and Gibbs (1980), and Stahura, Huff and Smith (1978) corroborates these findings. But what is the nature of the relationship between percent black and robbery?

Christopher Dunn (1980), in his review of crime area research, emphasizes that this relationship can*not* simply be explained in terms of the low socioeconomic status of area residents since "the race composition of areas has effects on crime distribution which are independent of socioeconomic status" (p. 17).[33] While the persistence of this finding has elicited explanations consistent with a wide range of criminological perspectives,[34] it is the interpretation of social ecologists that is most

---

[31]Flango and Sherbenou's (1976) urbanization variable was one of six extracted factors the authors used as independent variables in a multiple regression analysis. They found that urbanization explained 40.8% of the variance in robbery in larger cities (n = 153), but only 12.6% of the variance in smaller cities (n = 687).

[32]The black/white dichotomy presented in this section ignores other minorities, in particular citizens of Spanish descent. The data on other groups were not available from the 1977 County and City Data File. Thus, the white category is actually a residual category including all other posssible minorities. Clearly, this limits our understanding of ethnicity in areas of the country (e.g., percent Mexican-American in Houston) where blacks are not the dominant minority group. See Chilton, Chapter 6 for a discussion of this volume.

[33]See Christopher S. Dunn, "Crime Area Research," Chapter 1, in Georges-Abeyie and Harries (1980, p.5-25). According to Dunn, we cannot explain away the ethnicity effect in terms of socioeconomic status.

[34]In particular, Georges-Abeyie (1981) provides a discussion of the following criminological explanations of this correlation (e.g., labelling theorists; conflict theorists; conservative criminologists, such as control theorists; the structural functionalists; and social ecologists). This is the author's typology of theory.

relevant to the present study. Georges-Abeyie (1981) summarized this perspective.

The above average rate of black criminality is in large part due to the fact that blacks reside in "natural areas" of crime, that is, blacks reside in the ecological complex demarcated by the following social, economic, psychological, cultural, and spatial factors:

(1) deteriorating or deteriorated housing
(2) limited or nonexistent legitimate employment and recreational opportunities
(3) anomic behavior patterns
(4) a local criminal tradition (which started prior to the duration of the current black ethnic group in residence)
(5) abnormally high incidence of transient or psychopathological individuals
(6) a disproportionate number of opportunities (due to mixed land use) to engage in criminal deviance or to develop subcultures that are extra-legal (criminal or quasi-criminal)
(7) an area where poverty and limited wealth is the norm rather than the exception. (p.99)

While this explanation cannot be fully examined using data from the present study, it should be emphasized that the ethnicity-robbery correlation reported here (i.e., for all cities, Beta = $-.46$; $p < .05$ with percent white as the indicator) was independent of a host of physical characteristics (including city size, density, overcrowding, housing style and type, opportunity, and commercial differentiation) as well as other population-compositional variables (including income, poverty, and education). This finding poses a serious challenge to the viability of the "natural area" explanation.

Moreover, when larger and smaller cities were examined separately, ethnicity was the most important factor explaining intercity variation in robbery rates. Since these "natural areas" are usually indentified in large urban settings, ethnicity should be less important than physical characteristics such as size when larger cities are examined separately. However, both city size and ethnicity were moderately correlated with the robbery rate in larger cities. Surprisingly, ethnicity is comparatively more important than city size (Betas = $-.48$ and .16, respectively) in smaller cities. While these findings give some credence to the arguments of compositional (nonecological) theorists, as noted earlier, this perspective has difficulty accounting for the persistence of the size-robbery correlation.[35] Thus, it should be clear that *both* offer incomplete explanations of the size-robbery and ethnicity-robbery correlations.

---

[35]The compositional (nonecological) position holds that this relationship will disappear once relevant population-compositional variables are controlled. One alternative explanation here is that inadequate measures of population composition preclude this type of comparison.

The limitations of both perspectives can best be highlighted by examining regional variation in these two ecological correlates of robbery. In the Northeast and South, both ethnicity and city size were the main determinants of variation in intercity robbery rates. However, city size was insignificant in the North Central region, while ethnicity was unimportant in the West. Neither perspective offers an adequate explanation for these findings by itself; thus it may be the *interaction* of both sets of factors which holds the key to understanding intercity variation in robbery rates.

Implications

It is recognized that cities are constantly in change; but to change cities we must first understand the nature of the interactions which are taking place.[36] Clearly, to understand the causes of intercity variation in the rate of property crime, we must first understand *how* the essential characteristics of cities (e. g., physical and population-compositional variables) affect crime rates in these areas. The present study contributes to our knowledge of this process, by emphasizing the complex nature of these interactions. Perhaps most importantly, it is now apparent from the results of the size-specific analyses reported here that aggregation bias has plagued much of the existing research on cities and crime. Indeed, specific policy recommendations consistent with the findings reported here are premature since possible *intra*crime variation has yet to be explored. This is the next logical step in ecological research on cities and crime; homogeneity cannot be assumed.

Acknowledgments: This is a revised version of a paper presented at the 1983 annual meeting of the American Society of Criminology, Denver, Colorado. The author would like to thank Robert Sampson, University of Illinois, Champaign-Urbana and Dawood Farahi, Kean College of New Jersey, for their review and comments.

---

[36]For an excellent compendium of research on cities and the change process, see Walton and Carns (1973).

6
Age, Sex, Race, and Arrest Trends for 12 of the Nation's Largest Central Cities

ROLAND CHILTON

The demographic composition of most central cities in the United States has changed dramatically over the past 2 decades. Although their metropolitan areas have grown, many older central cities have been losing population since at least 1960. These population losses have been accompanied by changes in ethnic—especially racial—and age composition. Since the age-specific nature of most serious offenses is well known, we would expect such changes to have an impact on crime and arrest rates. The general conclusions of earlier efforts to assess the impact of demographic changes on U.S. crime rates was that the youthful population was decreasing and that this decrease in the proportion of young people would probably result in decreases in crime. (Chilton & Spielberger, 1971, Ferdinand, 1970; President's Commission, 1967; Sagi & Wellford, 1968)

However, most of these attempts to assess the importance of a changing age structure for increases in crime have involved the use of arrest data aggregated for the United States, a data set with some serious limitations. The major disadvantage of these national arrest counts is that the agencies providing information changed from year to year. For example, the number of urban police agencies providing arrest data in 1960 was 2,460; the number providing such data in 1980 was 8,487. (Federal Bureau of Investigation 1961; 1981) Since it is not possible to extract data for the same places at two or three points in time from published arrest data, assessing the impact of demographic changes on a selected set of cities— using unpublished Uniform Crime Reporting (UCR) data—seemed more useful than attempting to adjust the national estimates for this purpose.

Working with data from the same set of cities not only increases comparability but also permits the identification of anomalous or unexpected situations which may be important in understanding the trends reported. For example, when data for Boston were examined, it appeared that changes in age composition contributed little to the increased arrests in the city from 1960 to 1980—until race was included as a classifying variable.

When an age-specific analysis was conducted by race and gender, it suggested that over 58% of the increase in total arrests was understandable in light of increases in the number of individuals in specific age-sex-race categories. (Chilton, 1983), The Boston analyses also revealed the reason for the failure of a general age-specific analysis to identify the impact of changes in age composition on arrest counts. The *increase* in the number of people in the 15- to 29-year-old age group occurred in part as a result of the changing racial composition of the city. The 15- to 29-year-old white population increased from 1960 to 1980 by 11,000; the 15- to 29-year-old nonwhite population increased by 36,000.

In the analysis reported here, procedures similar to those used to analyze the Boston data were used to examine the impact of changes in the age, gender, and racial composition for 12 of the nation's largest central cities. Sets of these cities constitute 9 of the 10 largest cities in the United States in 1970 or 1980. Cities with the 10 largest populations in 1970 were New York, Chicago, Los Angeles, Philadelphia, Detroit, Houston, Baltimore, Dallas, Washington, D.C., and Cleveland. By 1980, Washington and Cleveland had dropped to 15th and 17th, respectively, and were replaced by San Diego and Phoenix. Data from 9 of these cities are used in the full analysis. Boston, which was the 16th largest city in 1970, was added to this set as a large, older northeastern city.

Unfortunately, New York, the largest central city in this set, had to be excluded from the analysis because the number of arrests of persons in specific racial categories were not reported for New York City until 1977. This situation would make any estimate of the impact on arrests of New York's changing racial composition extremely speculative. We know that the city's white population decreased by about 27% from 1960 to 1980 and that its nonwhite population increased by approximately 92% over this same period. However, there is no dependable way to estimate white and nonwhite arrests in the city prior to 1977, and therefore no way to examine changes in the racial characteristics of persons arrested from 1960 to 1980.[1]

Washington, D.C. and Detroit also present special problems for

---

[1]These increases are approximate because a 1980 change in census procedures for classifying persons of Spanish Origin by race in 1980 produced white and nonwhite figures which were not comparable with census figures prior to 1980 (Census, 1983a; 1983b). The 1980 Census figures used in this analysis have been adjusted to make them comparable with 1960 and 1970 white and nonwhite counts. For a detailed discussion of the 1980 Census change and its impact on white and nonwhite rates, see Chilton and Sutton (in press).

analysis. Since, in both cities, the number of arrests decreased from 1960 to 1980, the question is not how much of the increase in arrests can be explained by demographic changes but how much of the *decrease* in arrests is explained by such changes. Therefore, data for these cities were examined separately, suggesting that 70% of the *decrease* in arrests in Detroit was due to the decrease in the white population and decreasing white arrest rates. In Washington, less than 1% of the total decrease in arrests is attributable to decreases in the white population. White arrest rates actually increased, producing an increase of white arrests of 1,873. Therefore, almost all (99%) of the total decrease in arrests in Washington can be attributed to decreases in nonwhite arrest rates. Some of the remaining 10 cities listed in Table 6.1 also present unique patterns, but overall decreases in arrests were not reported for any of them and counts of arrests by age, race, and gender were available for all.

Data and Method

Unpublished Part I arrest counts for the twelve cities examined below were provided by the UCR Section of the FBI.[2] From 1960 to 1973 police agencies submitted annual reports of the number of arrests made for 27 specific offenses. After 1973, these agencies submitted monthly reports which were then converted to annual totals by the UCR staff. The counts in these reports were made by gender within specific age categories. With the exception of a few years, data were provided for these cities for each year from 1960 through 1980. Population data for each of the cities was obtained form U.S. censuses for 1960, 1970, and 1980 (Census, 1963;1973;1982).

The basic procedure used in the age-specific analyses presented below involves the computation of arrest rates for specific age-sex-race categories for 1960 and 1980. The 1960 rate is then used with 1980 population data to compute the expected number of 1980 arrests. The explicit research question in such an analysis is: How many arrests would we expect in 1980 if the arrest rates for specific categories of people did not change but the number of people in these categories did? The goal of the effort is to estimate the proportion of the total increase (or decrease) in arrests which might be explained by changes in the composition of the population.[3]

---

[2]Part I arrests for 1960 through 1980 included homicide, rape, robbery, assualt, burglary, larceny, and motor vehicle theft.

[3]The categories examined are those created by age, sex, and race classifications. Population counts for the cities studied—for specific age groups—for nonwhite males, nonwhite females, and white females are provided in census publications.

TABLE 6.1. Contribution of Specific Age Categories to Changes in Part I Arrests from 1960 to 1980 for 10 of the Largest Central Cities in the United States[a]

Age	1960 arrests		1960 % of population	1980 arrests		1980 % of population	Change 1960–1980	% of total increase
	No.	%		No.	%			
−15	18,829	18	28.0	26,341	12	21.6	7,512	6.3
15–19	30,175	29	6.6	78,410	35	9.0	48,235	40.7
20–24	16,978	16	6.4	47,502	21	10.7	30,524	25.8
25–29	11,616	11	6.5	29,335	13	9.9	17,719	15.0
30–34	9,350	9	7.0	17,394	8	7.9	8,044	6.8
35–39	6,810	7	7.3	8,779	4	5.9	1,969	1.7
40–44	4,233	4	6.8	5,467	2	4.9	1,234	1.0
45+	6,736	6	31.4	9,930	4	30.1	3,194	2.7
Total	104,727	100	100.0	223,158	99	100.0	118,431	100.0

[a]The cities are Baltimore, Boston, Chicago, Cleveland, Dallas, Houston, Los Angeles, Philadelphia, Phoenix, and San Diego.

Analysis

Tables 6.1 and 6.2 illustrate the utility of the procedure when information for 10 of the largest cities in the country is aggregated for Part I arrests. In Table 6.1 we can see that people in specific age categories are over-represented in the arrest data—in relation to their numbers in the general population. Arrests of 15- to 19-year-olds in these 10 cities constituted roughly 29% of the arrests for 1960, but those in this age group made up less than 7% of the population in that year. By 1980, they constituted almost 9% of the population and 35% of all arrests. In fact, 41% of the total increase in arrests can be attributed to increased arrests of persons in this age group. Arrests of persons in the larger 15- to 29-year-old age category account for almost 82% of the increase in arrests from 1960 to 1980.

Table 6.1 does *not* indicate how much of the total increase in arrests can be expected as a result of the increase in the number of 15- to 29-year-olds in these cities. Table 6.2 contains the results of a more systematic age-specific analysis of changes in the combined Part I arrests for these 10 cities from 1960 to 1980.

The expected arrests (col. 7) are computed by dividing the arrests for 1960 by the populations for that year and multiplying the result by the

---

Arrest counts for the same cities and age groups are provided by the UCR program for males and females. A separate UCR count of arrests by race is available which is not subclassified by age and gender, reflecting the procedure used to collect the data. (See footnote 5)

1980 population. This answers the following question: If the 1960 age-specific rates had remained constant, how many arrests could be expected in each age category in 1980? The expected change (col. 8) is the expected arrests minus the 1960 arrests; The observed change (col. 9) is the actual 1980 arrests minus the 1960 arrests. Where the expected change is negative, none of the observed increase is explained by change in the number of people in that category.

Moreover, in summing the expected changes—to see what percentage of the total increase in arrests might be explained by changes in the age composition—it is important to total only the positive numbers. When this is not done, expected decreases in some categories will reduce the effect of expected increases for other categories. In Table 6.2, the total expected increase was 33,547 Part I arrests, the total observed increase 118,431—suggesting that 28% of the total increase might be expected as a result of increases in the number of people in the 15- to 34-year-old age categories. Since the size of the other age groups decreased, none of the total increase in arrests can be explained by increases in the population of those under 15 or over 34 years old.

To determine the percentage of the total increase explained by a population increase in a specific age category, the expected increase for that category is divided by the total observed increase. The percentage of the observed increase attributable to an increased rate of arrest for a specific age group is the observed increase minus the expected increase for that age group divided by the total observed increase. In Table 6.2, for example, of the observed increase in arrests of 15- to 19-year-olds, 12,548 were expected given the increase in the number of individuals in the group from 870,000 to 1,231,000. This suggests that approximately 11% of the total increase in arrests is explained by this increase in population. Another 30% (48,235 minus 12,548, or 35,687) must be attributed to an increase in the arrest rate for this age group.

Using this procedure, an examination of Table 6.2 suggests that the changing age composition of this set of cities will explain at most 28.3% of the total increase in arrests.[4] It also indicates that 27% of this total increase, (almost all of the 28%) is explained by increases in the number of persons over 15 and under 30, although another 55% of the total increase can be attributed to the increased *rates* of arrest for the three age groups 15-19, 20-24, and 25-29.

---

[4]The 28.3% figure masks differences in the importance of a changing age composition between northern and southwestern cities. For five cities in the southwest and west this figure is 76.3%. However, for the five cities in the midwest and east it is 7.9%. Other differences between these two sets of cities are presented in the text.

TABLE 6.2. Age-Specific Analysis of Part I Arrests 1960 to 1980 for 10 of the Largest Central Cities in the United States[a]

Age	1960 population	1960 arrests	1960 rate[b]	1980 population	1980 arrests	1980 rate[b]	Expected arrests	Expected change	Observed change
-15	3,689,310	18,829	510	2,966,813	26,341	888	15,142	-3,687	7,512
15-19	869,291	30,175	3,471	1,230,783	78,410	6,371	42,723	12,548	48,235
20-24	847,885	16,978	2,002	1,470,804	47,502	3,230	29,451	12,473	30,524
25-29	860,628	11,616	1,350	1,358,921	29,335	2,159	18,342	6,726	17,719
30-34	916,051	9,350	1,021	1,091,836	17,394	1,593	11,144	1,794	8,044
35-39	957,898	6,810	711	812,787	8,779	1,080	5,778	-1,032	1,969
40-44	897,549	4,233	472	676,446	5,467	808	3,190	-1,043	1,234
45+	4,135,887	6,736	163	4,139,791	9,930	240	6,742	6	3,194
Total	13,174,499	104,727	795	13,748,181	223,158	1,623	132,512	27,785	118,431

Total observed increase   118,431
Total expected increase[c]   33,547
Percent explained   28.3

[a]The cities are Baltimore, Boston, Chicago, Cleveland, Dallas, Houston, Los Angeles, Philadelphia, Phoenix, and San Diego.
[b]Number per 100,000 population.
[c]The sum of the positive values in the expected change column.

The age-specific analysis shown in Table 6.2 is somewhat misleading in that it masks known differences in male and female age-specific rates. When these are taken into account, by an examination of the contribution of males and females to the 1960-to-1980 arrest increases, we find that the increase in arrests of 15- to 29-year-old males accounts for 67% of the total increase. (See Table 6.3.) The increase in arrests of 15- to 29-year-old females accounts for another 15% of the total increase. For all ages combined, the increase in arrests of women and girls for this set of cities accounts for 20% of the total increase in arrests and the increase in arrests of men and boys accounts for 80%. Since these percentages can be computed from information in Table 6.3, no separate table is presented.

The age-specific analysis shown in Table 6.3 suggests that just over 30% of the total increase in arrests can be explained by the increase in the number of people in the 15- to 29-year-old age group. Most of the expected increase, almost 33,000 arrests or almost 28% of the total increase, can be attributed to the increase in the population of 15- to 29-year-old males. Another 3,000, or roughly 2.5% of the total, can be attributed to the increase in 15- to 29-year-old women, in the population. Table 6.3 also shows a narrowing of differences in arrest rates for men and women. Although there continue to be considerable differences in such rates, the arrest rate for 15- to 29-year-old women, which was less than 1/10 of the male rate in 1960, increased to 1/6 (17%) of the male rate by 1980.

With 65% of the total increase in arrests in this set of cities being the result of increases in arrests of persons classified as nonwhite, we can assume that a reasonable proportion of the total increase was the result of an increase in the number of 15- to 29-year-old nonwhite males. To estimate this number, and the number of people in other age-sex-race categories, male and female arrests by race for specific age groups were estmated on the assumption that the proportion of nonwhite arrests in each age-sex category was the same as the proportion of all arrests classified as arrests of nonwhite persons.[5]

Table 6.4 shows the results of the age-specific analysis by race and sex which was undertaken using this assumption. It suggests that 53% of the

[5]To estimate nonwhite arrests within the specific age-sex categories used, each age-sex arrest count for a city was multiplied by the proportion of all arrests in that city which were classified as arrests of nonwhite individuals. Age- and sex-specific white arrest counts were estimated using the same procedure. The procedure assumes, for example, that the proportion of arrests of 15- to 19-year-old males classified as nonwhite was the same as the proportion of arrests of 30- to 35-year-old males classified as nonwhite, and that both are equal to the proportion of all arrests so classified.

TABLE 6.3. Age-Specific Analysis by Sex of Part I Arrests from 1960 to 1980 for 10 of the Largest Central Cities in the United States[a]

Age and gender		1960 population	1960 arrests	1960 rate[b]	1980 population	1980 arrests	1980 rate[b]	Expected arrests	Expected change	Observed change
−15	M	1,864,922	16,872	905	1,508,026	22,315	1,480	13,643	−3,229	5,443
15–29	M	1,259,878	53,125	4,217	2,041,756	132,308	6,480	86,094	32,969	79,183
30–44	M	1,352,353	17,701	1,309	1,266,848	25,687	2,028	16,582	−1,119	7,986
45+	M	1,925,324	5,737	298	1,812,534	7,416	409	5,401	−336	1,679
−15	F	1,824,388	1,957	107	1,458,787	4,026	276	1,565	−392	2,069
15–29	F	1,317,926	5,644	428	2,018,752	22,939	1,136	8,645	3,001	17,295
30–44	F	1,419,145	2,692	190	1,314,221	5,953	453	2,493	−199	3,261
45+	F	2,210,563	999	45	2,327,257	2,514	108	1,052	53	1,515
Total		13,174,499	104,727	795	13,748,181	223,158	1,623	135,475	30,748	118,431

Total observed increase   118,431
Total expected increase[c]   36,023
Percent explained   30.4

[a]The cities are Baltimore, Boston, Chicago, Cleveland, Dallas, Houston, Los Angeles, Philadelphia, Phoenix, and San Diego.
[b]Number per 100,000 population.
[c]The sum of the positive values in the expected change column.

increase in arrests from 1960 to 1980 can be explained by increases in the number of people in specific age-sex-race categories. Forty-four percent of this increase in arrests was the result of an increase of 61% in the nonwhite population. Nine percent was the result of an increase in the 15- to 29-year-old white population; another 26% of the increase can be attributed to increases in white arrest rates. This suggests that the changing racial composition of this set of cities and their relatively high nonwhite arrest rates are more important as explanations of the increase in arrests than the overall change in age composition or the increase in rates of arrest of women. The increase in the rates for white females will account for only 8% of the 118,000 increased arrests and the increased rates for nonwhite females only another 8%. However, another 4% of the increase in arrests can probably be attributed to increases in specific nonwhite female population categories.

The examination of changes in estimated arrest rates by race and gender simultaneously suggests that the arrest rates for nonwhite women were higher than those for white women in 1960 and that although the rates for white women increased more rapidly from 1960 to 1980, the arrest rates for nonwhite women were still higher than those for white women in 1980. Moreover, the changing racial composition of this set of cities means that there were also fewer white women in the population in 1980 than there were in 1960, while the number of nonwhite women increased sharply.

This is important because it suggests that as the number of young nonwhite women in central cities increases, we may observe sharper increases in female arrest rates in these cities than we would if there were no change in racial composition. At this point it is not possible to know how these changes have affected national trends. However it seems likely that any analyses of the changing involvement in crime by women which assumes that these increases are distributed equally across racial categories will produce misleading results. Moreover, the extent to which increases in arrest rates of women are influenced by large increases in the arrests of young nonwhite women will be important for interpretations of such increases.

It is also important to note that there appear to be major regional differences in age-specific arrest trends. If the set of 10 cities examined above is divided into those in the midwest or east and those in the southwest, we find that 15- to 29-year-olds account for most of the total increase in both cities (79-83%). However, the changing age-sex-race composition of cities in the southwest accounts for 78% of the observed change in these cities while the changing age-sex-race composition of the five cities in the midwest and east accounts for only 35% of the total increase.

Moreover, increases in nonwhite arrests constitute 79% of the total increase in arrests in the five cities in the midwest and east—in contrast

TABLE 6.4. Age-Specific Analysis by Race and Gender of Part I Arrests from 1960 to 1980 for 10 of the Largest Cities in the United States[a]

Age, race, gender	1960 population	1960 arrests	1960 rate[b]	1980 population	1980 arrests	1980 rate[b]	Expected arrests	Expected change	Observed change
NM −15	499,667	8,784	1,758	632,675	13,562	2,144	11,122	2,338	4,778
NM 15–29	272,284	27,507	10,102	677,207	78,614	11,609	68,414	40,907	51,107
NM 30–44	300,444	9,566	3,184	389,932	15,036	3,856	12,415	2,849	5,470
NM 45+	304,856	3,104	1,018	473,440	4,290	906	4,820	1,716	1,186
NF −15	507,202	979	193	621,261	2,201	354	1,199	220	1,222
NF 15–29	322,778	2,911	902	736,026	13,032	1,771	6,638	3,727	10,121
NF 30–44	331,289	1,460	441	469,266	3,350	714	2,068	608	1,890
NF 45+	320,639	538	168	614,604	1,385	225	1,031	493	847
WM −15	1,365,255	8,088	592	875,351	8,753	1,000	5,186	−2,902	665
WM 15–29	987,594	25,618	2,594	1,364,549	53,694	3,935	35,396	9,778	28,076
WM 30–44	1,051,909	8,135	773	876,916	10,651	1,215	6,782	−1,353	2,516
WM 45+	1,620,468	2,633	162	1,339,094	3,126	233	2,176	−457	493
WF −15	1,317,186	978	74	837,526	1,825	218	622	−356	847
WF 15–29	995,148	2,733	275	1,282,726	9,907	772	3,523	790	7,174
WF 30–44	1,087,856	1,232	113	844,955	2,603	308	957	−275	1,371
WF 45+	1,889,924	461	24	1,712,653	1,129	66	418	−43	668
Total	13,174,499	104,727	795	13,748,181	223,158	1,623	162,767	58,040	118,431

Total observed increase 118,431
Total expected increase[c] 62,896
Percent explained 53.1

[a]The cities are Baltimore, Boston, Chicago, Cleveland, Dallas, Houston, Los Angeles, Philadelphia, Phoenix, and San Diego.
[b]Number per 100,000 population.
[c]See last note for Table 6.2. In addition, the expected increase for each line is limited to the observed increase for that line.

with 44% for the five cities in the southwest. There are also differences
between these two sets of cities in the proportion of the total change
which can be attributed to increases in white arrest rates—21% for the
cities in the midwest and east and 56% for cities in the southwest.

Nevertheless, the suburbanization and segregation patterns observed
in midwestern and eastern cities are likely to be repeated in the
southwest. In fact, while the central city white populations of the five
southwestern cities did not decrease from 1960 to 1980—as they did in all
five northern cities—the increases in the nonwhite populations in Dallas
and Los Angeles exceeded the increases in the white population. In Los
Angeles the white population increased by 131,000, the nonwhite by
357,000. The combined white population of the cities of the southwest
increased by 1,088,000 from 1960 to 1980 while the nonwhite population
increased by 934,000. By 1990, most of these cities may present trends
similar to those shown for the cities in the midwest and east, where the
white population *decreased* by 2,269,000 while the nonwhite population
increased by 821,000.

Discussion

In 1980 the set of 10 cities examined above constituted less than 7% of the
total U.S. population and 10% of the total number of Part I arrests
reported by age. However, preliminary analysis of 40 of the nation's
largest central cities suggests that the pattern found here will be
substantially reproduced when arrests and demographic changes in this
larger set of cities are analyzed.[6] To the extent that detailed analyses
support this expectation, it appears that the changing racial composition
of the nation's largest cities has produced a substantial part of the
increased crime observed in urban areas since 1960. Changes in age
composition are still important but in most central cities they appear to
be the result of changes racial composition. Changes in the conduct of
women and girls also appear to explain some of the observed increase.
However, these changes also appear to have been heavily influenced by
the racial composition of these central cities.

The overrepresentation of young people in criminal activity is well
known as is the fact that men and boys are disproportionately involved.
However, the patterns produced when changes in age gender, and race
are examined simultaneously have received less attention.[7] The results

---

[6]These preliminary analyses, for example, suggest that between 40% and 50% of
the increased arrests in these 40 cities can be attributed to the increased arrest of
nonwhite males.

[7]Notable exceptions to this are studies by Block and Zimring (1973), Block
(1975;1977), and Hindelang (1981).

presented above suggest that for many central cities the change which has had the greatest impact on arrest counts has been the changing racial composition of these cities.

Among the most plausible interpretations of this trend are the persistently limited economic circumstances of young nonwhite men and women and the changing family arrangements of those remaining in large areas of many central cities.[8] Both of these situations may be contributing to socialization processes which are more likely to result in criminal conduct than those produced by more stable family situations and more comfortable economic circumstances. Although it seems extremely unlikely that similar patterns will be found for the suburban areas around the same cities, an important next step is the development of age-specific analysis by race and sex for the noncentral city areas of these Standard Metropolitan Statistical Areas. A more complete understanding of the trends involved will also require analyses of specific types of arrests.

These results are also important for theories developed to explain systematic variation in criminal involvement with age. The best known of these was proposed by David Greenberg in 1979. Although in his concluding comments, Greenberg overstates his case by suggesting that all teenagers have a "common, if temporary, relationship to the means of production"(1979, p. 215), in his critique of other delinquency theories he recognizes that this relationship is not the same for all categories of young people. His statement that "those whose opportunities for lucrative employment are limited by obstacles associated with racial and/or class membership will have less reason to desist from illegal activity than those whose careers are not similarly blocked" (1979, p.210) leads him to suggest that "rates in given offense categories should decline more rapidly for whites . . . than for blacks . . ."(p.211). The suggestion is not quite consistent with the age distributions of arrest rates constructed from data used in this analysis, perhaps because the social and economic circumstances of the white population remaining in many central cities has worsened in the past 2 decades.

Greenberg's treatment of male and female differences in delinquency involvement is not entirely clear. However, in general, his discussion suggests that girls will probably steal less because they will perceive less need to steal than boys (1979, p.198). Although he does not explicitly discuss differences between white and nonwhite males or white and nonwhite females, his suggestion of understandable differences in rates by race and gender make his assertion that there is a single juvenile class seem forced.

---

[8]For discussions of the social and economic status of central city black populations, see Bureau of the Census (1978) and Wilson (1980).

His statement that juveniles cannot be routinely assigned to the class of their parents makes sense. Nevertheless, young people cannot be routinely assigned to the same class either. The economic situation of most young men is still different from that of most young women. More importantly, as Greenberg recognizes, the economic situation of most nonwhite young people, especially nonwhite males, is dramatically different from that of white young people—male and female.

However, perhaps the major limitation of Greenberg's presentation as a theoretical analysis of age distribution and criminal involvement is its focus on juveniles. Age-specific analyses of data for all age groups suggests that many forms of crime continue into adulthood. Although some rates peak at 15 and 16, others, such as homicide and assault, peak at 21 and are relatively high for 20- to 24-, and 25- to 29-year-olds. For some offenses,differential involvement by people in older age categories are striking. Therefore, the restriction of discussions of age variation in involvement in crime to teenagers unnecessarily truncates the age distribution of criminal activity.

The implication of Greenberg's sweeping assertion is that different categories of young people will have roughly the same rates of arrest. Although the age-specific analyses conducted for this chapter fail to support this possibility, they provide more support for Greenberg's emphasis on the importance of age variation for theories of crime than they do for Hirschi and Gottfredson's equally sweeping assertion that "the age-crime relation is invariant across sex and race" (1983, p.556). Although the meaning of invariance is unclear in their discussion and perhaps is misleading because they treat differences in level as an exception (p.556), they go on to suggest that with some modifications, "the form of the age curve of person offenses [approximates] that for property offenses" (p.558).

When age distributions for specific offenses are examined for specific race-sex categories for the cities studied for this chapter, regional variations in the age distribution appear which suggest that for cities in the northeast and midwest the curve of the age distribution is flatter for nonwhite arrests—especially nonwhite female arrests—than it is for white arrests. In these cities, the estimated larceny arrest rates for nonwhite women remain relatively high for 20- to 24- and 25- to 29-year-old women. The rates for white women in these age groups are sharply lower than the rate for the 15- to 19-year-old white group.

Given the limitations of the data used (i.e., the need to estimate the white and nonwhite age-sex-specific arrest counts) and the preliminary nature of this comparison of age distribution curves, these findings are merely suggestive. However, this analysis does indicate that much more analysis of the age distribution of offense data and arrest data is necessary before it can be said with any confidence that "the age

distribution of crime is invariant across social and cultural condition"
(Hirschi and Gottfredson, 1983, p. 554).

Part of the confusion on this issue may be produced by the use of self-
report data to analyze age distributions. Self-report studies have almost
always been limited to school-age young people, thus truncating the age
distribution of the population under study. Moreover, these studies lose
dropouts and many truants and have frequently been limited to male
respondents. Equally important for this discussion is the fact that self-
report studies have sometimes had so few nonwhite respondents that they
can be said to truncate the social-class distribution of the populations
they are intended to represent.[9]

Perhaps the most important implication of the analyses presented
above is the support it appears to provide for perspectives stressing the
importance of social-class and economic factors in the production of
criminal activity. Although socialization also appears to be important (as
indicated by the differences among specific race and sex categories) it
appears more likely that the economic situations of millions of nonwhite
men and women is one of the best explanations for increases in crime
and arrests in these cities. At a minimum, the longstanding and
worsening economic situation of millions of young nonwhite males, in a
society which places great emphasis on consumption, would appear to
make additional crime likely. Whatever interpretation appears most
convincing at this stage, additional studies of demographic changes and
their impact on arrests are almost certain to identify trends with which
contemporary theories of crime must come to grips.

Acknowledgments: This is a revised version of a paper presented at the
1983 annual meeting of the American Society of Criminology, Denver
Colorado. I am indebted to the Uniform Crime Reporting Section of the
FBI for the provision of unpublished arrest data and to the Graduate
School and the Computing Center of th University of Massachusetts for
financial support and computer time.

---

[9]Hirschi's (1969) analysis of self-reported delinquency data, for example, virtually
eliminates nonwhite respondents. In a footnote he indicates that "because of the
greater unreliability of Negro data, partly stemming from their generally low
verbal skills, the bulk of the analysis and the data presented in the remainder of
this work is restricted to whites". (p.79). The analysis of social class and
delinquency which preceded this note was also limited to white males—the girls
having been previously removed from the analysis.

7
Urban Crime Rates: Effects of Inequality, Welfare Dependency, Region, and Race

RICHARD ROSENFELD

If crime is to be explained from a sociological perspective, it should be viewed as a product of social organization. The two basic dimensions of social organization are *culture* and *social structure*. There are, in turn, two generic causal models of crime in sociology: a *cultural model,* which explains crime as a product of conformity to cultural or subcultural values, and a *structural model*, which explains crime as a product of structural discontinuity or disorganization.[1] Two contemporary variants of the structural model of crime may also be distinguished: *control theory* and *strain theory*. Control theory assumes that crime results from a breakdown in structural controls over behavior. Strain theory assumes that crime results from an anomic imbalance or contradiction between culture and social structure.[2]

This chapter derives empirical propositions from the two sociological models of crime and examines them with data on urban crime rates in the United States. A proposition is derived from strain theory linking variations in urban crime rates with relative deprivation. Control theory is investigated in an analysis of the effects of welfare dependency on urban crime. The cultural model is assessed in an analysis of regional and racial effects on violent crime. Some of the findings of the empirical analysis, including those concerning the connection between race and crime, call into question common theoretical assumptions and the results of recent studies in the literature on the structural and cultural sources of variation in aggregate crime rates. The theoretical implications of these

---

[1]It may be objected that there are at least two additional "models" of crime and deviance in sociology, the conflict and interactionist perspectives, and perhaps even one more, the functionalist theory of deviance. However, these perspectives are not strictly commensurate with the cultural and structural models because they do not intend to explain the causes so much as the *consequences* of deviance.

[2]See Rosenfeld (1984) for a detailed explication of each of these perspectives.

and other findings are considered in the conclusion of this chapter, and several avenues for subsequent investigation are suggested.

Data and Method

The unit of analysis employed in this study is the Standard Metropolitan Statistical Area (SMSA). The type of analysis is cross-sectional and the method is ordinary least-squares regression. The dependent variables are the index crimes reported in the Uniform Crime Reports (UCR) for SMSAs in 1970 (Federal Bureau of Investigation, 1971). The offense data are derived from police reports and are expressed as rates per 100,000 population. The findings and conclusions of this investigation are thus limited by the well-known validity and reliability problems affecting all studies which utilize "offenses known to the police."[3]

Independent variables are derived from data obtained from census and other sources as described below. Each subanalysis is based upon the total number of cases for which all requisite data were available.

Strain, Relative Deprivation, and Crime

Strain theory, of which Merton (1938) is the exemplar, holds that crime results when legitimate structural means are insufficient to attain culturally approved success goals. "Success," from this perspective, is not biologically or psychologically fixed, but culturally and historically variable. It follows that crime should be related to economic inequality rather than a poverty of means, to relative rather than absolute deprivation (see Coser, 1967, for an explicit connection between strain and relative-deprivation approaches to crime).

However, differential access to legitimate means is not, by itself, a sufficient cause of crime. Structural inequality or deprivation produces pressures to deviate under very specific and distinct cultural circumstances. Merton maintains that the relationship between "deprivation and crime" is high where there is great "cultural emphasis on monetary accumulation as a symbol of success," and low where there is not. For Merton, culture conditions the association between structural inequality and crime (Merton, 1938, p. 680-681).

---

[3]See the review in Decker, Schichor, and O'Brien (1982, p. 21-24). Some researchers have concluded that, in spite of their shortcomings, the UCR measures are fairly valid for purposes of intercity comparisons (e.g., Hindelang, 1974; Skogan, 1974). Other researchers have questioned this assumption, at least for certain of the index offenses (Booth, Johnson, and Choldin, 1977; Decker, Shichor, and O'Brien, 1982; O'Brien, Shichor, and Becker, 1980).

Two propositions may be derived from this discussion: (1) Crime rates should be more strongly associated with variations in inequality than poverty rates. (2) The relationship between crime and inequality should be maximized in the presence of strong aspirations for economic achievement. Both propositions receive support in recent empirical investigations of urban crime rates.

Several recent studies have found a relationship between income inequality and urban crime rates, many also reporting little or no relationship between poverty and crime after inequality is controlled (Blau & Blau, 1982; Braithwaite, 1979; Council on Municipal Performance, 1973; Danziger, 1976; Danziger & Wheeler, 1975; Jacobs, 1981; see, also, the review in Long & Witte, 1981). Moreover, Rosenfeld (1982) reports significant associations between several violent and property crimes and a "relative deprivation" variable (RD) which incorporates a measure of economic aspirations along with economic inequality. Because these findings are based upon the same data set used to test propositions from the other sociological perspectives on crime, and for ease of direct comparison, they are reproduced here.

Table 7.1 displays the effects of RD, in the form of standardized regression coefficients, upon the rates of seven index offenses for the 125 largest SMSAs in 1970. RD is defined as the product of the intensity of deprivation, the scope of deprivation, and the level of economic aspirations among poor families in the SMSA.[4] The intensity of deprivation is measured by the difference between the mean income of families below the poverty level and the mean income of all families in the SMSA. The scope of deprivation is measured by the percentage of families with incomes below the federal poverty level in 1969. Aspirations are measured by the ratio of median years of school completed by heads of poverty families to median years of school completed by all family heads. This measure assumes that the economic aspirations of low-income people will vary directly with their educational attainment vis-á-vis that of middle-income comparative referents (see Rosenfeld, 1982, p. 13-15, for a more complete description of and rationale for RD).

Table 7.1 also shows the effects of three additional variables on crime rates, employed as controls in this analysis: SMSA population size (POP), unemployment rate (UNEM), and regional location (REGION).[5]

---

[4]The intensity of deprivation may be defined as the degree of discrepancy or difference between *capabilities* and *expectations*. The scope of deprivation refers to the proportion of a population sharing some specified level of deprivation (see Gurr, 1970, p.59-91).

[5]Population totals are 1970 estimates from Federal Bureau of Investigation (1971). The unemployment measure is the percentage of the unemployed civilian labor force, taken from U.S. Bureau of the Census (1973). Regional location is a South-nonsouth dummy variable.

TABLE 7.1. Standardized Regression Coefficients and Coefficient of Determination for Relative Deprivation, Controls, and Crime (N = 125)

	Murder	Rape	Robbery	Assault	Burglary	Larceny	Motor vehicle theft
POP	.19*	.17**	.68*	.24*	.17*	.11	.37*
UNEM	−.14	.01	.00	−.04	.21**	.22**	−.09
REGION	.49*	−.04	.17	.42*	.10	−.07	−.17
RD	.27*	.52*	.06	.30*	.39*	.33*	.28**
R^2	.52	.30	.48	.46	.32	.20	.21

Note. POP = SMSA population size. UNEM = unemployment rate. REGION = regional location. RD = relative deprivation. Table adapted from Rosenfeld (1982: Table 4).
*$p \leqslant .01$. **$p \leqslant .05$.

The disproportionate concentration of crime in large cities is a long-standing criminological finding, often interpreted in terms of Wirth's (1938) classic discussion of urban heterogeneity, density, and anonymity (see, e.g., Skogan, 1979, p. 380-382). In light of the substantial body of theory and research on unemployment and crime (see Braithwaite, 1979; Long & Witte, 1981; Thompson, Sviridoff, & McElroy, 1981) it seems advisable to include a measure of unemployment in the present investigation. Finally, regional location is included for purposes of subsequent analysis of the thesis of a southern subculture of violence.

Controlling for population size, unemployment rate, and regional location, relative deprivation has significant effects on six of the seven index offenses. While the absence of an effect on robbery rates is puzzling, these findings are generally consistent with the proposition that crime is generated by economic inequality in the presence of high aspirations. Moreover, other findings show that the combination of aspirations with inequality has a stronger effect on crime rates than does inequality alone, consistent with strain-theoretical expectations (see Rosenfeld, 1982, p. 15). If the measure of relative deprivation employed in this study is a valid operationalization of Mertonian strain theory, there would seem to be considerable support for the theory at the aggregate level.

Control, Welfare Dependency, and Crime

Control theories locate the causes of crime and delinquency in the absence or weakening of social control (Hirschi, 1969; Kornhauser, 1978; Reckless, 1973). The breaking of the social bond or deterioration of internal or external constraints upon behavior "frees" the individual to deviate. From a control perspective, a basic function of social structure is to link culture with behavior. Individual behavior is socially controlled to the extent it is directed along culturally approved pathways. Two important institutional settings in which normative controls are implemented are the family and the labor market. If the control function of either of these institutions is seriously attenuated or disrupted, deviance and crime are likely to result.

The public provision of monetary assistance to poor families (welfare) has been criticized for undermining the control functions of both the family and labor market, and therefore for generating crime. Conservative critics of the "War on Poverty" charged that the "welfare explosion" of the 1960s was at least partially responsible for skyrocketing crime rates in American cities (see, e.g., Banfield, 1970; Wilson, 1975). More recently, a conservative writer has claimed that the expansion of the assistance rolls during the 1960s actually *reversed* ongoing improvements and brought about unprecedented levels of suffering, dependency, and pathology in urban poor communities (Gilder, 1981, p. 13). The conservatives maintain that welfare leads to crime by disrupting and breaking apart families and by weakening labor-market controls. Gilder claims that the increased availability of assistance resulted in "a virtual plague of family dissolution". Furthermore, because the availability of nonmarket incomes reduces reliance upon labor-market incentives, welfare contributes to the high labor-force withdrawal rates of teenagers (especially blacks), and therefore to high teenage crime rates (Gilder, 1981, p.14).

The conservative critique of welfare dependency has an interesting complement in recent radical analyses of American social policy. Gilder's argument concerning the impact of public assistance on labor-market controls is, in essentials, quite close to the Piven-Cloward thesis on state policy, public assistance, and labor-market functioning. While they have little to say about crime rates per se, Piven and Cloward (1971, 1982) propose that a crucial function of income maintenance and other social-welfare programs has been to weaken employer control and power over labor. However one radical analyst has explicitly linked welfare and urban crime rates: "One might even say that through AFDC, the federal government places its stamp of approval on both the fatherless inner-city family and the pursuit of crime as the solution to black men's unemployment problems" (Harris, 1981, p.131).

Despite their differences concerning crime causation, both the conservative and radical critiques of welfare policy predict that cities with high dependency rates should, other things being equal, also have high crime rates. The single existing study of the effects of public assistance on variations in SMSA crime rates (DeFronzo, 1983) focuses upon *levels* rather than rates of assistance. DeFronzo (1983) looked at the effects of the level of Aid to Families with Dependent Children (AFDC) payments upon crime rates among the 39 SMSAs for which 1970 cost-of-living data

TABLE 7.2. Standardized Regression Coefficients and Coefficient of Determination for Welfare Dependency, Welfare Eligibility, Controls, and Crime (N = 204)

	Murder	Rape	Robbery	Assault	Burglary	Larceny	Motor vehicle theft
POP	.21*	.29*	.65*	.23*	.25*	.15**	.36*
UNEM	−.12**	.15**	−.04	−.04	.23*	.27*	−.13**
REGION	.57*	.21*	.14**	.49*	.31*	.23*	.03
WELEL	.14**	.16	.04	.17**	−.02	−.17**	−.03
WELDEP	.20*	.11	.12	.10	.11	.03	.33*
R^2	.48	.18	.49	.35	.19	.13	.32

Note. POP = SMSA population size. UNEM = unemployment rate. REGION = regional location. WELEL = welfare eligibility. WELDEP = welfare dependency.
*$p < .01$. **$p < .05$.

were available. He found a *negative* relationship between benefit levels and the rates of homicide, rape, and burglary, controlling for income inequality, unemployment, racial composition, and other factors.

This chapter investigates the relationship between crime and assistance rates, as measured by the percentage of the poverty population receiving public assistance. Table 7.2 shows the effects of this measure of welfare dependency (WELDEP) on the seven index offense rates for the 204 SMSAs for which the requisite data were available. Controls are introduced for population size (POP), unemployment rate (UNEM), and regional location (REGION) (as previously described). The crime and population data are from Federal Bureau of Investigation (1971). The unemployment and welfare data are from U.S. Bureau of Census (1973). WELDEP is defined as the percentage of families with incomes below the poverty level receiving public assistance. Thus WELDEP is a measure of dependency and not simply a redundant measure of poverty. Table 7.2 also includes a separate measure of welfare *eligibility* (WELEL).

There is, not surprisingly, a moderate tendency for SMSAs located in states with lenient AFDC guidelines to have higher rates of welfare dependency than those located in more restrictive states.[6] However, neither welfare variable has a strong or consistent effect upon crime rates. Dependency shows a small but significant effect upon murder rates and a moderate effect upon motor-vehicle theft. The latter is somewhat

---

[6]r = −.39. WELEL is derived from the index of restrictiveness of state AFDC eligibility guidelines reported in Campbell and Bendick (1977, p. 85-86). Each SMSA was assigned the index value of the state in which it is located. The more restrictive a state's guidelines, the higher its score on the index, thus accounting for the negative correlation between WELDEP and WELEL.

_545555

surprising in light of DeFronzo's conclusion that, owing to both the highly organized nature of the offense on the one hand, and youthful "fun and excitement" quality on the other, assistance should have little effect upon motor-vehicle theft (DeFronzo, 1983, p.132). Eligibility restrictiveness has small significant effects on murder, assault, and larceny rates. However, in the cases of murder and assault, these results are the *opposite* of what would be expected on the basis of the conservative critique of welfare policy. Consistent with DeFronzo's (1983) findings for benefit levels, there is a slight tendency for cities with relatively lenient welfare eligibility rules to have lower rates of murder and assault than those with more restrictive rules.

Overall, however, the present investigation provides only weak support for arguments stipulating a welfare-crime connection, positive or negative. While these results are provisional and should be replicated under alternative specifications,[7] they do indicate that the effect of welfare dependency on crime has probably been exaggerated by both conservative and radical critics of welfare policy. They provide no support for conservative proposals to substantially restrict welfare eligibility, at least in so far as such efforts are justified as a means to reduce moral decay and crime.

Culture and Crime

The cultural model holds that crime results from conformity. An important application of the model is the "subculture of violence" thesis, which argues that much criminal violence results from conformity to subcultural norms which encourage and support violent and aggressive behavior (Wolfgang & Ferracuti, 1967). Two variants of the subculture of violence thesis are considered in this paper. The first is the Hackney-Gastil hypothesis that accounts for high rates of violent crime in the American South in terms of distinctive regional cultural orientations (Hackney, 1969; Gastil, 1971). The second is the idea of a "black violent contraculture" developed by Curtis (1975) and elaborated by Silberman (1978). The empirical consequences of each of these applications will be

---

[7]Thus, it could be argued that including welfare dependency and eligibility restrictiveness in the same regression model washes away the effects of the latter on crime rates, since these effects should operate through variations in dependency, which have been controlled. However, if WELDEP is removed from the model and the effects of WELEL are recomputed controlling only for POP, UNEM, and REGION, the results are essentially the same. A small and barely significant positive effect remains for Assault, and a small and significant negative effect remains for Larceny. No significant effect remains for Murder ($\beta = .07, p = .24$).

examined against those derived from alternative structural approaches to violent crime.

Southern Violence

The thesis of a Southern subculture of violence was developed to explain why rates of violent crime, murder and violent assault in particular, have historically been greater in the states of the Confederacy than elsewhere. There is more violence in the South, it has been argued, because a distinctive complex of values developed there which triggers and channels the expression of violent behavior. The historical sources for this violent subculture are said to include defeat in the Civil War, accompanied by a "siege mentality" and defensive Southern pride and honor (Hackney, 1969), the institution of slavery, and the lengthier frontier experience of Southern settlements (Gastil, 1971). Whatever its sources, the violent-value complex is assumed to have persisted beyond its original structural moorings.

The cultural explanation of Southern violence has been questioned by investigators who claim that rates of violence are higher in the South because there is greater structural deprivation and inequality there, and not because distinctive Southern values foster violence (see, e.g., Blau & Blau, 1982; Braithwaite, 1979). The competing claims have been evaluated at the aggregate level according to the assumption that structure explains violence to the degree that, when structural variables are controlled, the association between region and crime disappears, and culture explains violence to the degree it does not. The structural explanation has been upheld in certain investigations (e.g., Blau & Blau, 1982; Erlanger, 1974; 1976; Loftin & Hill, 1974), and the cultural explanation in others, notably Messner (1982; 1983).

If the presence of regional effects after structural variables are controlled is taken as evidence for the cultural approach to Southern violence, the present study lends support to the cultural position. Table 7.1 shows that, with population size, unemployment rate, and a measure of relative deprivation controlled, substantial regional effects upon murder and assault remain. Significantly, in both cases the regional effect is larger than the effect of relative deprivation. The absence of significant regional effects for nonviolent offenses, or for the violent offense of rape, provides further substantiation for the cultural argument. The effect of regional location is specific to precisely those offenses predicted to have subcultural causes.

Additional structural variables will have to be included in subsequent analyses of the regional subculture-of-violence hypothesis before alternative explanations can be conclusively rejected. However, these findings, together with Messner's (1982; 1983) results for homicide, shift the burden of proof back to those who would continue to argue that regional variations in urban violent crime rates are due wholly or primarily to poverty or inequality.

Race and Crime

"In the end," writes Silberman (1978:117), "there is no escaping the question of race and crime." The inescapable question to which Silberman refers concerns the possibility of a cultural component to black crime in the United States that is not fully reducible to structural deprivation or inequality. Silberman's (1978) discussion of race and crime leans heavily on the idea of a "violent black contraculture" advanced by Curtis (1975) to account for the high rates of criminal violence in cities with large black populations. The contraculture, which emphasizes physical toughness, sexual exploitation, shrewdness, and thrill-seeking arose and is sustained, Curtis argues, as an adaptation to racial oppression and economic marginality. However, in spite of its ultimate structural determinants, the contraculture promotes violent and aggressive responses among the young ghetto males who adhere to it more-or-less independently of variations in poverty or racial inequality. At the aggregate level of analysis, then, the violent contraculture thesis would predict the persistence of an association between a city's racial composition and violent-crime rates, after measures of racial deprivation and inequality are controlled.[8]

This proposition is examined in the present investigation. It should be noted that a recent study employing data and measures similar to those used here concludes that there is little or no evidence for theories of violent crime which posit a distinctive culture of violence among blacks (Blau & Blau, 1982). The researchers base their conclusion on the following generalization from their data: " . . . once inequalities and two other conditions [population size and percent divorced] are controlled, racial composition accounts for little additional variation" in rates of murder and assault among the 125 largest SMSAs (p. 126). In fact, however, the data presented by Blau and Blau do not support their conclusion. The effect of percent black on the murder rate ($\beta=.36$) is substantially larger than that of any other variable they examine, including measures of intraracial income inequality ($\beta=.22$) and inter-

---

[8]Curtis (1975) provides support for the use of racial composition as an aggregate-level indicator of violent contraculture. Noting "agglomeration effects" on the transmission of contraculture values in urban ghetto areas, he suggests that the size of the black population is an important demographic determinant of "contracultural takeoff" (p. 36). He goes on to propose multicity studies of race and violent crime which investigate "differential outcomes as a function of relevant population size, proportion, and the like" (p. 36).

TABLE 7.3. Standardized Regression Coefficients and Coefficient of Determination for Racial Composition, Controls, and Crime (N = 125)

	Murder	Rape	Robbery	Assault	Burglary	Larceny	Motor vehicle theft
POP	.05	.17**	.62*	.13	.16**	.13	.41*
UNEM	−.14	.05	.07	−.15	.13	.18	.00
RD	.22*	.45*	−.08	.45*	.53*	.40*	.15
BL	.55*	.06	.37*	.22**	−.10	−.17	.01
R^2	.56	.30	.53	.41	.32	.21	.20

Note. POP = population size. UNEM = unemployment rate. RD = relative deprivation. BL = percent black.
*$p \le .01$. **$p \le .05$.

racial inequality ($\beta=.25$). The effect of racial composition on the assault rate is also greater than those of the inequality measures (Blau & Blau, 1982, p. 124). The Blau's data, if not their conclusions, are consistent with Messner's (1983) findings for a larger sample of SMSAs.

The present study examines the contraculture thesis with the same methods and logic of analysis used by Messner (1983) and Blau and Blau (1982), but with a greater number and variety of racial-deprivation and inequality variables to serve as controls. The analysis proceeds by examining the effects of racial composition on urban crime rates controlling, first, for a general measure of relative deprivation (RD) and then for a series of measures of racial deprivation, discrimination, and inequality.

Table 7.3 shows the effect of percent black (BL)[9] on violent and property crime rates, controlling for relative deprivation (RD), population size (POP), and unemployment rate (UNEM), for the 125 SMSAs for which the requisite data were available. The data reveal significant racial effects on murder, robbery, and assault, no significant effects on property offenses, and no effect on rape. With the exception of the latter, these findings conform to the pattern expected on the basis of Curtis' violent contraculture thesis.

An alternative explanation of these findings from the structural perspective would hold that the relationship between race and violent crime is interpreted by racial deprivation. To investigate this possibility, three measures of racial deprivation were introduced into the analysis: the black poverty rate (BLPOV), median years of school completed by black family-heads (BLEDUC), and the black male unemployment rate

[9]Computed from data in U.S. Bureau of the Census (1973).

TABLE 7.4. Standardized Regression Coefficients and Coefficient of Determination for Racial Composition, Racial Deprivation, and Crime (N = 79)

	Murder	Robbery	Assault
BLPOV	.08	−.54*	.20
BLEDUC	−.04	.20	.18
BMUNEM	−.26*	.03	−.19
BL	.45*	.61*	.33**
R^2	.46	.31	.19

Note. BLPOV = black poverty rate. BLEDUC = median years of school completed by black family-heads. BMUNEM = black male unemployment rate. BL = percent black.
*$p < .01$. **$p < .05$.

(BMUNEM).[10] Table 7.4 shows the effects of racial composition on murder, robbery, and assault rates with these deprivation measures controlled. Significant racial effects remain in each case. Moreover, racial deprivation, at least as reflected in poverty, educational, and employment indicators, has surprisingly weak effects on crime rates. Strikingly, in the two instances where there is any significant deprivation effect at all, the effect is the *opposite* of that predicted by structural theory. High poverty and unemployment rates are associated with low robbery and murder rates, respectively.

A possible objection to the structural variables considered thus far is that they measure absolute deprivation, whereas previous research, as noted, has indicated a relationship between *inequality* and crime. However, similar results emerge when inequality measures are substituted for the deprivation variables. Table 7.5 displays the effects of racial composition on murder, robbery, and assault rates, controlling for three measures of racial inequality: (1) the difference between the median income of black families and the median income of all families in the SMSA (RACEGAP); (2) the black male unemployment rate divided by the total male unemployment rate (RACEUNEM); and (3) residential segregation by race (RACESEG).[11]

---

[10]From U.S. Bureau of the Census (1973) for the 79 SMSAs for which all requisite data were available.

[11]The income and unemployment measures were constructed from data from U.S. Bureau of the Census (1973). The segregation data are tract-based indexes of dissimilarity for SMSAs in 1970 (reported in Van Valey, Roof, & Wilcox, 1977). The analysis is based upon the 196 SMSAs for which all requisite data were available.

TABLE 7.5. Standardized Regression Coefficients and Coefficient of Determination for Racial Composition, Racial Inequality, and Crime (N = 196)

	Murder	Robbery	Assault
RACESEG	.14*	.39*	.05
RACEGAP	.06	.01	.02
RACEUNEM	−.14*	−.08	−.12**
BL	.66*	.29*	.51*
R^2	.55	.29	.31

Note. RACESEG = residential segregation by race. RACEGAP = difference between the medium income of black families and the medium income of all families in the SMSA. RACEUNEM = the black male unemployment rate divided by the total male unemployment rate. BL = percent black.
*$p < .01$. **$p < .05$.

Racial composition has significant effects on the three violent crimes, while the effects of the inequality variables are weaker and inconsistent. The dollar gap between blacks and whites has no independent influence on crime rates. Unemployment inequality has significant effects on murder and assault, however they are in the opposite direction of that predicted by structural theory. The performance of racial segregation is somewhat better. Indeed, of the six structural variables included in this analysis, segregation is the only one which shows significant and predictable effects on violent crime. Segregation is positively associated with rates of murder and robbery, although not with rates of assault. In no case, however, can it be said that the effect of race on crime is fully explained by racial segregation.

Conclusions

The empirical results of the present study may be summarized as follows:

1. The investigation finds mixed support for the structural model of crime.
   a. There is substantial support for the propositions, derived from strain theory, that (i) crime rates are more strongly associated with inequality than with poverty, and (ii) the relationship between inequality and crime is maximized in the presence of high achievement aspirations.
   b. There is a weaker support for the control-related proposition that welfare dependency is positively associated with crime.
2. The investigation finds strong support for the cultural model of crime.

 a. Regional effects on violent-crime rates persist after structural factors are controlled.
 b. Racial effects on violent crime persist after structural factors, including measures of racial deprivation and inequality, are controlled.

The provisional nature of these findings bears repeating. They are intended to produce guidelines for further research and not firm conclusions regarding the complex interplay of culture, social structure, and crime. Additional research is required utilizing alternative measures of theoretical constructs and model specifications. The relative-deprivation measure employed in this study should be tested with different units of analysis (e.g., nation states) and on time-series as well as cross-sectional data. The difficult question of the *differential* effects of inequality on crime rates must also be tackled. All crimes are not affected equally by variations in the intensity and scope of deprivation among American cities. For example, robbery is apparently not affected at all. Why are robbery rates not responsive to variations in economic inequality when, say, rape and assault rates are? The problem here is not that relative deprivation was found to be associated with violent crime, for there is theory and research to support such a relationship, but that deprivation is associated with some violent offenses but not others.

Similar considerations apply to the investigation of control theory undertaken here. Control theory is not invalidated by a finding of weak effects of welfare dependency on crime, because dependency is only one of many plausible indicators of control. Subsequent investigations might, for example, include legal sanctions as indicators of formal social-control. They have been omitted from the present analysis primarily because of the difficulty of operationalizing system-response variables at the SMSA level.

Perhaps most important, we did not examine the possible indirect effects of welfare policy on crime. In so far as the effect of dependency operates through family dissolution, family variables should be incorporated in subsequent analyses, and indirect as well as direct effects on crime should be investigated. The effects, if any, of family dissolution are likely to be quite complex. A review of the relevant literature finds little evidence for a direct causal connection between "broken homes" and delinquency (Rosen & Neilson, 1978). The conventional assumption of a differential connection of broken homes with female delinquency has also been questioned and qualified (Datesman & Scarpitti, 1980). Harris' (1981) discussion of crime and welfare dependency, however, posits a mediating role for the family. As such, it is consistent with recent proposals to inject the family into theory, research, and policy aimed at the "underclass" (see Kelly, 1982). This approach conceives of the lower-class family as more-or-less capable of exercising "resource sharing/

acquisition" and "stress mediation" functions for its members. To the extent that these functions are maintained, the family protects members from the pathogenic effects of long-term economic deprivation (Kelly, 1982).

If, additionally, welfare dependency is argued to reduce labor-force participation among teenagers, participation and age variables should be investigated, and the connections among welfare, secondary labor markets, and crime clarified (see Myers, 1978). Finally, if, as Gilder (1981) implies and Harris (1981) states explicitly, welfare dependency produces high crime rates specifically among urban blacks, then racial composition needs to be included in future studies of welfare and crime, and race-welfare interaction effects explored.

The cultural model of violent crime was upheld, or at any rate could not be rejected, by this investigation. This does not mean that structural factors were found to be inconsequential in accounting for variation in rates of violent offenses. Table 7.3 shows that relative deprivation is significantly associated with rates of murder, assault, and rape when racial composition (a proxy measure of "violent contraculture") as well as other factors are controlled. Table 7.1 shows significant relative-deprivation effects for several violent and property offenses when regional location (a proxy for a Southern "subculture of violence") and other conditions are controlled. In the context of recent theory and research, however, what is significant about these findings is not the presence of structural effects, but the persistence of *cultural* effects with structural conditions controlled. In the face of studies such as Blau and Blau (1982), Loftin and Hill (1974), and Parker and Smith (1979), the finding, at the aggregate level, of any cultural effect at all is anomalous.

Implications

A general problem for future research is to reconcile the differences between these and other findings obtained at different levels of analysis. The existence of violent subcultures has not been established in survey research on value orientations (see Ball-Rokeach, 1973), and, of course, investigators must be extremely cautious and tentative when inferring cultural causation from aggregate relationships. Part of the discrepancy in findings at different levels of analysis may well be conceptual in nature. Perhaps the essence of the violent subculture, like other delinquent subcultures, is not so much a held-in-common value preference for violence as a "shared misunderstanding" concerning the violent preferences of others (see Matza, 1964). Such an interpretation would link cultural and social-disorganization approaches to violent crime.

Acknowledgments: This is an abridged and revised version of a paper presented under the title "Culture, Social Disorganization, and Urban Crime Rates" at the 1983 annual meeting of the American Society of Criminology, Denver, Colorado.

Part III The Impact of Ecological
Factors on Decision
Making and Policy in the
Criminal Justice System

8
Person-Environment Interactions in the Prediction of Recidivism

STEPHEN D. GOTTFREDSON AND RALPH B. TAYLOR

Introduction

The purpose of the research reported here is to aid in the understanding and prediction of criminal recidivism. The general research question may be stated quite simply: By considering the socio-environmental context into which an offender is released after a period of incarceration, can we improve upon recidivism predictions which are based solely on personal characteristics of the offender?

Despite the "obviousness" of the research question, surprisingly little is known about it. In a recent review of attempts to predict violent and aggressive behavior, Monahan (1981) repeats a call made earlier by Shah (1978): The role of situational factors must be addressed if we are to improve our ability to predict behaviors of the sort under consideration. Similarly, a recent report by the National Research Council of the National Academy of Sciences (1981) suggests that research on the social and environmental factors contributing to criminal behavior is necessary and missing.

Although the research problem appears straightforward, it is conceptually, methodologically, and practically complex. Three research traditions are relevant: the risk-prediction tradition, ecological/areal research on delinquency, and studies of neighborhood and community dynamics.

The Risk-Prediction Tradition

For the past half-century, considerable effort has been expended in the development of statistical devices designed to aid criminal justice decision makers, and many jurisdictions now use such devices. Most of this development has involved the prediction of parole performance (see reviews in Gottfredson, 1967; Gottfredson and Gottfredson, 1979, 1980, 1985; Mannheim & Wilkins, 1955; Simon, 1971) or, more recently, performance on bail release (Freed & Wald, 1964; Goldkamp, 1979;

Goldkamp & Gottfredson, 1979, 1985; Gottfredson, 1974). Typically, the predictive power of risk-screening devices is not great (cf. Simon, 1971; Gottfredson & Gottfredson, 1979), although it is usually better than simple base-rate prediction.

Among the major methodological problems of behavioral prediction are issues such as the relative efficiency of "clinical" versus "actuarial" or statistical methods of prediction (Dawes, 1977, 1979; Dawes & Corrigan, 1974; Einhorn & Schact, 1980; Gough, 1962; Meehl, 1954); the relative efficiency of different actuarial approaches (Gottfredson & Ballard, 1964; Gottfredson & Gottfredson, 1979; Gottfredson, Wilkins, Hoffman, & Singer, 1974; Simon, 1971; Solomon, 1976; Van Alstyne & Gottfredson, 1978; Wilbanks & Hindelang, 1972); the base-rate problem (Meehl & Rosen, 1955); the criterion problem and associated measurement issues (Gottfredson, 1967; Schmidt & Witte, 1979; Waldo & Griswold, 1979); and problems of the reliability of predictor measures and resultant stability of the models or equations developed (Cronbach, 1960; Cureton, 1967; Gottfredson, 1967; Gottfredson & Gottfredson, 1979). These concerns, albeit neither exclusive nor exhaustive, do include the major assessment issues which must be addressed by researchers interested in the prediction of behavior.

The concept of "risk environments" is central to our research. Suppose our investigation indicates that prediction can be improved if the environment to which an offender is to be released is known, and the risk and support features of that environment can be assessed. From a purely empirical perspective, it would appear desirable to incorporate these "environmental" variables into prison release decisions. As a practical matter, however, this may not be desirable—and potentially could raise legal challenges (Underwood, 1979).[1] It is important, therefore, to stress that concerns of policy and practice must not be confused with concerns of theoretical and empirical scientific advance. The research that we have been pursuing is, we believe, of considerable theoretical importance; yet without careful attention to policy issues, it may have limited immediate practical application. Each concern is vital, but in different arenas. We hope eventually to provide advances to both.

Ecological/Areal Research

Investigations in this area have differed substantially with respect to their conceptual bases. This brief review focuses on three relatively distinct research traditions.

Human ecology. The "human ecological" perspective (Park, 1916) developed from the ecological framework successfully used in biology.

---

[1] A more practical application, therefore, may be in assessing supervision needs once a release decision has been made.

According to this view, concepts of "ecological niches," "environmental competition," and so on, have counterparts in criminology. Processes of urban change and development are seen to be such that particular locales are differentially influenced by large-scale economic and "subsocial forces" (Michelson, 1970), resulting, for some locales, in social disorganization. Thus, Shaw and McKay (1942) observed that delinquency rates were high in areas where physical deterioration was also high, and that delinquency varied inversely with distance from the city center (see also Thrasher, 1927). It appeared that delinquency showed the same "spatial pattern" as did many other pathologies (Faris & Dunham, 1939).[2]

Later work replicated and extended these findings, associating delinquency and/or crime rates with socioeconomic status (Harries, 1979, provides a comprehensive review). Factors related to housing (crowding, vacancies, substandard conditions), employment (unemployment rates, welfare rates), and family characteristics (percent of single-headed households) were found to covary with delinquency rates.

Considerable debate developed concerning whether these results reflected socioeconomic status or "anomie" (Gibbons & Jones, 1975; cf. Merton, 1957). Lander (1954) argued for the latter, and subsequent replications appeared to support this contention (Bates, 1962; Bordua, 1958; Chilton, 1964; Polk, 1957). Gordon (1967; see also Hirschi & Selvin, 1967) later demonstrated that results of several statistical methods had been miscalculated or that the techniques themselves had been misused (often in subtle ways) in much of this research. Thus, Gordon concluded that "when all of these errors are taken into account, it turns out that the association between delinquency and socioeconomic status is quite unambiguously very strong."[3]

Many sociological (as opposed to biological or psychological) theories of crime causation deal largely with the social environment and its interaction with individuals or groups (Cloward & Ohlin, 1960; Gibbons & Jones, 1975; Hirschi, 1969; Matza, 1969; Merton, 1957; Reckless, 1973). Not surprisingly, the ecological/areal research findings have been important to much of this theory construction. Of course, the association between crime or delinquency rates and social characteristics, although strong and consistent, is (a) not perfect, (b) more than likely operates

---

[2]For a review of human ecology, see Morris (1957) or Michelson (1970); for a review of delinquency research from an ecological perspective, see Baldwin (1975, 1979); for a critique, see Taylor (in press).

[3]It is important to note, however, that this does not deny the possible co-occurrence of anomie and disorganization. Further, it is not clear whether anomie, socioeconomic status, or both, is most closely related to social disorganization. Finally, Gordon's conclusions are not supported by recent work based on self-report methods (Hindelang, Hirschi, & Weiss, 1981).

through several (often unspecified) mediating factors (cf. Hirschi & Selvin, 1967; Willie, 1967), and (c) if specified, are difficult to measure adequately (Meier, 1982; Greenberg, Rohe & Williams, 1984).

One suggestion of how this relation functions was proposed by Shaw and McKay (1942), and tested by Maccoby, Johnson and Church (1958). Shaw and McKay suggested that the distribution of socially maladjusted youth was relatively uniform throughout an urban area, but that modes of controlling (or of failing to control) children varied from community to community. Maccoby, Johnson, and Church's research supported this hypothesis, and aggregate-level research has identified similar relations between intra- and inter-household "cohesion" factors and delinquency (Dentler & Monroe, 1961; Glueck & Glueck, 1950; Hirschi, 1969; Quinney, 1964; Schmid, 1960).

Positive local forces. A very different conceptual base for understanding spatial variation in crime and delinquency can be found in work that focuses on neighborhood and community qualities. Burgess (1925) suggested that there were three types of social forces operating at the neighborhood level: ecological, cultural, and political. This framework has been used by others to investigate criminal outcomes, and a compelling demonstration of its utility is Warren's work on riots (Warren, 1969, 1977, 1978). He suggested that neighborhoods vary on three dimensions: (1) the extent of attachment to local community; (2) the degree of informal social exchange among neighbors; and (3) "vertical" ties to the larger community. Warren observed that riot behavior was elevated in neighborhoods lower in social exchange and attachment, and that "counter-riot" activity was elevated in neighborhoods in which neighboring linkages were extensive. Apparently, such neighborhood-level attributes may help preserve social order.

Situational factors. A third stream of research has been concerned with the micro-level situational correlates of crime, violent behavior, and recidivism. This work has dealt with physical environmental factors that may create "opportunities" for crime (see Taylor, 1982; Taylor, Gottfredson, & Brower, 1980 for reviews), and social, employment, and family-related stressors. This situational approach, as articulated by Monahan and Klassen (1982), includes family-related stressors (e.g., Straus, 1980), peer-related stressors (e.g., Davies, 1969), and job-related stressors (Cook, 1975). Following recent trends in personality psychology, Monahan and Klassen suggest that attention to situational variables may greatly enhance power to predict crime-related outcomes, and that current devices may be overly constrained by a "trait" approach.

The Neighborhood Perspective

Areal socio-demographic factors are correlated with crime-related outcomes, and these relations obtain even when individual-level characteristics are statistically controlled (Sampson, 1983b). If we are to understand fully the *nature* of these relations, we need conceptual tools to help in deciding (a) the appropriate areal unit(s) to study, (b) which ecological variables theoretically are important, and (c) how these best can be measured. Thus, we have a geographical problem, a conceptual problem, and a measurement problem. We believe that use of the concept of *neighborhood* may prove useful in providing the needed framework.

The concept has been used widely and contradictorily over the last half-decade. It has been proposed as a fundamental planning unit (Dahir, 1947; Rohe & Gates, 1981), attacked as segregationist (Issacs, 1948), and treated as a polity (Crenson, 1983; Frederickson, 1972) and as a basic arena for primary (Cooley, 1902; Gans, 1962) and secondary (Mann, 1970) ties. Not surprisingly, debate has emerged regarding differential use of the term (see Taylor, 1982, for a review; see also Hunter, 1974, 1978; Keller, 1968; Suttles, 1968, 1972; Wellman & Leighton, 1979).

We see three advantages to using a neighborhood perspective for the selection of socio-environmental variables for our purpose. First, neighborhood may be a clearly bounded spatial unit. Second, as defined in Baltimore (Goodman & Taylor, 1983; Taylor, Brower & Drain, 1979), neighborhoods have substantial ecological integrity, and the areas are recognized by insiders and outsiders alike. Finally, there has been extensive attention given to their social and psychological functions (Popenoe, 1973; Warren, 1977).

Thus, use of the neighborhood concept can help solve the geographic and conceptual problems concerning socio-environmental character-istics we raised earlier. We expect that three classes of neighborhood-related variables will be associated with crime-related outcomes. The first is the nature and extent of *local social ties* (Fischer *et al.*, 1977; Granovetter, 1973; Mitchell, 1969). It is through local ties that informal sanctions or controls are asserted (Warren, 1963). Thus, pressure to conform with local norms may be mediated by local social networks. Second, local ties are important for instrumental outcomes such as finding a job (Granovetter, 1974) or a place to live, as well as use of local services (Froland & Pancoast, 1979).[4]

The second class of neighborhood variables are those concerned with *attachment to locale* (Gerson, Stueve & Fischer, 1977; Shumaker & Taylor, 1983; Warren, 1978) that is, the extent to which residents are involved in local events, and feel positively about and responsible for what goes on in the neighborhood.

The third relevant class of neighborhood variables is the extent, location, and distribution of *local services*. Conceptions of "community"

---

[4]Of course, the "controlling network" in the neighborhood in which a potential offender lives may have less of a deterrent effect if offenders' targets are outside of the neighborhood.

(Froland & Pancoast, 1979; Gerson et al., 1977; Warren, 1963) rely heavily on these notions of the location and type of local service institutions. A reasonable hypothesis is that some local services and community elements may prove supportive (e.g., presence of local churches, places of employment, social service agencies, job location agencies, etc.), while others may pose a risk (bars, liquor stores, concentrations of other offenders, etc.) to released offenders.

Propositions Based on the Literature Reviewed

This brief review of three research traditions relevant to the potential impacts of community environments on offenders released from a period of incarceration suggests a number of propositions which we have found useful in guiding our research. First, it is clear that statistical risk-screening devices do provide a useful adjunct to the correctional decision-making process. Although the power of such devices traditionally has been low, prediction usually is above the base rate, and is better than that based solely upon clinical assessments.

Second, it is clear that given the nature and availability of present predictor and criterion information, we are unlikely to see advances in predictive power based simply on the use of different statistical approaches. The most sophisticated and the simplest statistical methods result in devices of comparable predictive power. Rather, we are much more likely to advance our predictive ability through careful attention to the data themselves. Thus, a third proposition is that increases in predictive utility are likely to be realized through better and more careful measurement, particularly of recidivism itself.

A fourth proposition, and one which is supported by considerable empirical evidence, is that areal socio-economic and socio-demographic factors are related to delinquency rates. Perhaps of more importance, however, is a fifth proposition: that socio-environmental context, independent of socio-economic or demographic factors, appears likely to influence delinquency rates and post-release adjustment. If this is so, our reading of the literature suggests a sixth hypothesis: meaningful and ecologically valid geographic or areal units are needed to assess and understand the relations between socio-environmental variables and the crime-related outcomes of interest (e.g., delinquency, recidivism).

Two final propositions are that the concept of neighborhood can help to define the requisite ecologically valid geographic units, and that the neighborhood concept itself suggests three classes of contextual variables (nature and extent of local social ties, attachment to the locale, and potentially supportive or criminogenic facilities) that should be related to recidivism.

These propositions have formed the basis for the research in which we are engaged, and about which this paper presents preliminary findings. In the course of our investigation, we have developed several data bases: an offender data file, a neighborhood assessment file, a criterion data file, and limited information from the 1970 and 1980 censuses.

Methods[5]

Offender Data File

Information concerning criminal history, current offense, social history, demographic characteristics, and performance after release from imprisonment was obtained for the approximately 500 subjects of this study in June and July of 1981. Variables of interest were selected to include those which had shown predictive promise in past research on recidivism (Gottfredson & Gottfredson, 1979). Offenders studied were all those released from a period of incarceration in state institutions to any of 90 randomly-sampled Baltimore neighborhoods over a 2-year period. Double-blind intercoder reliability checks resulted in coefficients for items ranging from 1.00 to .78, and averaging .91.

All offenders released to our sample of neighborhoods between October 1978 and October 1980 were assessed in terms of follow-up in January 1982. Variables of interest were chosen to reveal as much as possible about the outcome of the offender's release, that is, not only whether there was a re-arrest, but also the nature of that occurrence (date, seriousness, and if known, disposition). Federal Bureau of Investigation rap sheets provided the data, and intercoder reliability coefficients for items ranged from .99 to.85, and averaged .94.

Environmental On-Site Assessment

A random sample of 90 Baltimore City neighborhoods (38% of all neighborhoods in Baltimore) was selected for study.[6] Subsequently, a 20% random sample of the blocks (defined as both sides of a street-face), with a minimum of four blocks in small neighborhoods, was chosen for on-site assessment by teams of trained raters. A total of 1,102 blocks, with an

---

[5]Detailed information concerning methods can be found in Gottfredson and Taylor (1982). Information on the environmental assessment methods can be found in Taylor, Shumaker and Gottfredson (in press).

[6]Almost all of the Baltimore City population lives in 236 recognized neighborhoods. These were defined by Taylor, Brower and Drain (1979) in a manner which recognized the ecological integrity of these areas. Subsequent analysis (Taylor & Talalay, 1981) provided support for the ecological integrity of the neighborhoods as defined.

average of over 12 blocks per neighborhood, was assessed using a standardized checklist.

Attributes were included on the checklist if prior empirical or theoretical work suggested that those elements were relevant to crime, crime-related outcomes, or social disorder. Attributes assessed included aspects of the street (e.g., number of dwellings, percent residential vs. commercial street frontage), appearance (e.g., graffiti, litter, vacant housing), land use (e.g., industrial, service, etc.), and social climate (e.g., group size and sex of people "hanging out"). Interrater reliability (of items and of scales which subsequently were developed) was assessed using the intraclass correlation (Shrout & Fleiss, 1979). Most items had acceptable block-level reliability (r(ic) > .60), and all items and scales retained for further analysis had excellent reliability at the neighborhood level (r(ic) > .90).

Measurement Issues

Perhaps the most important variable in a prediction study such as this is the criterion or outcome variable. Several problems with outcome variables commonly used in parole prediction research have been noted in the literature (Blumstein & Larson, 1971; Gottfredson & Gottfredson, 1979; Waldo & Griswold, 1979). These include: (1) the validity of available data as a measure of release outcome; (2) the inability of dichotomous success/failure criteria to capture the full range of post-release adjustment (and statistical difficulties inherent in the use of a dichotomous criterion); (3) the confounding effect of "time at risk" when comparing experiences of offenders who have been in the community for varying lengths of time; and (4) differing error rates depending upon the nature of the criterion chosen (e.g., arrest, conviction, or incarceration).

Seriousness

A major development in the measurement of recidivism has been the effort to improve upon simple success/failure outcomes through assessment of the seriousness of criminal acts. Efforts to measure the seriousness of crimes date from Thurstone (1927), and replications suggest that these judgments remain remarkably stable over time (Coombs, 1967; Krus, Sherman & Krus, 1977). Others, using similar methods, have developed more comprehensive schemes (Gottfredson, 1980; Rossi, Waite, Bose, & Berk, 1974; Sellin & Wolfgang, 1964). Post-release crimes of offenders in this study, both at arrest and later disposition, were recorded using a modification of the scale developed by Gottfredson (1980), resulting in (at least) a rank ordering of offenses.

Successes all received the same value on this outcome-zero, the lowest rank. Failures yielded a distribution from 1 to 60.[7]

Time at Risk

The problem of varying time at risk has been addressed in many ways. Those comparing the success rates of different groups have developed sophisticated methods to adjust for differences in time at risk among groups (Stollmack & Harris, 1974; Turnbull, 1977). When a measure of the success of each individual offender is required, however, the problem is different. The most common method of standardizing follow-up time for offenders released at different times has been to take the shortest follow-up period as the common denominator for all offenders. In our study, offenders were released over a 2-year period, and follow-up data were obtained for all offenders 14 months after the release of the last offender. To standardize in the traditional manner would have meant ignoring any offenses committed more than 14 months after each offender's release date. Obviously, this would involve ignoring information available for offenders released earlier, and also could have resulted in cohort effects. Further, although many offenders do recidivate within a year after release, substantial proportions recidivate later (Bercochea, Himelson, & Miller, 1972).

We decided upon a little-explored method of adjusting time at risk for our sample of offenders. The method allows us to use all the information available for each offender, while simultaneously controlling for time-at-risk differences. A variable that measured the months between the release date of each offender and the end of our follow-up period was calculated and used as an independent control variable to partial for variation in post-release performance that could be attributed to differences in time available. Any remaining variation can then be attributed to other offender characteristics or the environmental variables (or, of course, to error).[8]

---

[7]The least serious crimes are offenses such as trespassing and littering: the most serious are assaults and murders. For all practical purposes, the scale approximates interval-level qualities.

[8]Statistically controlling variation in time available is not a perfect solution to the problem of equating offenders released at different times. If it is true that different release cohorts have different characteristics, we would expect our "time available" variable to be correlated with those characteristics. Because of this interrelatedness, the control variable could be given "credit" for accounting for variance that is actually better accounted for by the related characteristics. However, using the control variable technique will allow us to assess directly whether time available is related to other characteristics, and the implications of any interrelatedness can then be considered.

Time Free

Another consideration is that not all offenders actually were free for the length of time available to them. Failures were rearrested, and in most cases, reincarcerated upon arrest or later at conviction. This information is interesting, however, and we explored its use not as a control, but as an outcome measure. It can be argued that the offenders who recidivate after several years are more successful than offenders who commit new crimes shortly after release. Both are failures, but the offender who had a longer successful adjustment may (in some sense) be considered less of a failure than the other. The third outcome criterion we used, then, is time free. Successes have no value on this variable, since they were not rearrested during our follow-up period (i.e., time free is equal to time at risk—our control variable). Analyses involving this outcome will tell us if we can predict what kinds of offenders, in what types of environments, will offend quickly.

Time Free and Seriousness

Finally, we experimented with a complex outcome variable that used information concerning the seriousness of post-release crime (if any) as well as time free to commit crime. We combine the seriousness score and time free variables to create this fourth criterion measure. (Again, successes are not considered in analyses using this criterion.) Failures were given a score equal to the seriousness score of their crime divided by their time free in months. Thus, a shorter time free raised an offender's score on this criterion, as did a more serious crime.[9]

Scales Based on On-Site Assessments

To reduce items from the on-site assessments, and as a check on the external validity of items, the environmental variables were correlated with average 1979–1981 neighborhood-level crime rates.[10] Environmental variables that consistently correlated in the hypothesized direction with crime rates were retained for further analysis. Subscales were developed to reflect particular environmental influences on social control. For example, since prior research has suggested that formation of cohesive

---

[9]The question of what ratio of seriousness to time free constitutes the best single index of success can not be answered on the basis of this or previous research.

[10]Since we were interested in assessing attributes of neighborhoods that could promote or inhibit criminal activity, crime rates were viewed as reasonable measures to use in a preliminary test of item validity. The 3-year average was used to meliorate effects of extreme variability over time often observed for crime rates calculated for small areas.

groups and informal social control are inhibited in areas of high levels of street and foot traffic, as well as in areas of high housing density, scales reflecting these were constructed.

Subscales and items that correlated with crime rates were subjected to principal components analyses to further reduce the dimensionality of the environmental measures. Inclusion of socio-demographic variables indicated that neighborhood racial composition was independent of dimensions based on the environmental assessments (i.e., the racial composition measures formed a separate factor). The final analysis we chose to use was based on a 67-neighborhood principal components analysis of on-site assessments alone.[11]

The first component, accounting for 34% of the variance, reflected general neighborhood decay, or, to use the terminology of Hunter (1978; also Lewis & Salem, 1981), social and physical incivilities. Neighborhoods with a high score on this dimension were characterized by the presence of graffiti and litter, vacant houses, and groups of males "hanging out." A general look of decay may signify that area residents are unable or unwilling to maintain their community; thus, the community may be less cohesive and more vulnerable to criminal activity. The second component (13% of the variance) reflected residential versus nonresidential land use. Neighborhoods with a high score on this dimension were characterized by the presence of commercial, industrial, or institutional land use, high automobile and foot traffic, and vacant lots.

Analytic Strategy

In seeking to identify the separable or unique contributions of time available in which to recidivate, offender and environmental characteristics, and the interactions of persons and places, we used analysis of covariance (by regression) methods (Cohen & Cohen, 1975).[12] Since time available was our control variable, it was entered on the first step in each analysis. Optimal clusters of offender-characteristic variables were entered on the second step, the environmental-decay scale was entered on the third step, and offender-characteristic X environmental factor interactions were entered on the fourth step. Thus, one may think of the

---

[11]No offenders were released to 23 of the neighborhoods originally sampled.

[12]Regression analyses are reported even for dichotomous outcomes for purposes of comparability. We are well aware of the limitations of Ordinary Least Squares (OLS) regression in such situations, and of advantages of other methods, such as logistic regression. Given the base rate of our sample, however, we are not seriously disadvantaged through use of simple regression methods.

proportion of variance explained by offender characteristics to represent the "main effect" for personal characteristics net of time available in which to fail. Similarly, results reported for the environmental scale represent the "main effect" contribution of environmental characteristics, net of time available and the personal characteristics.

Inclusion of interaction terms in regression equations is a simple—but sometimes cumbersome—process. One difficulty is that the possible number of interaction terms increases dramatically as variables are added to the equation. In the present case, this difficulty was meliorated through use of "clusters" of offender characteristics (e.g., representing criminal history, social history, financial need and dependency, etc.) and by the fact that we were using a single scale representing environmental incivilities.[13] However, inclusion of interaction terms usually results in a second problem. Since these terms are created from independent variables which are already included in the regression equation (in the usual case), the interaction term(s) and the predictor (main effect) variables often are highly correlated. Although this has no deleterious effect on the principal question at hand—the assessment of the statistical significance and magnitude of increments in variance explained (cf. Allison, 1977)—it may render some model parameters (e.g., regression coefficients) unstable. To err on the side of conservatism, we will not consider detailed specification of models involving interaction terms, and will limit concern to the provision of estimates of the relative contributions (increments in R^2) of offender characteristics, environmental characteristics, and the interactions of these, to the prediction of recidivism.

Preliminary Findings[14]

Tables 8.1 and 8.2 summarize results of these analyses. Table 8.1, which addresses the dichotomous arrest/no arrest criterion and the seriousness score criterion described earlier, is based on all cases for which requisite information was available. Table 8.2, which summarizes findings relative to the time free and the complex time free/seriousness criteria, is based on those members of the sample who in fact were arrested during the follow-up period (for successes, time free and time available—our control variable—are totally confounded).

---

[13]Theoretically, we are assuming that this scale stands as a proxy for social disorganization or social decay.

[14]All analyses discussed are based on arrests as a criterion, since disposition information was missing for many cases.

TABLE 8.1. Regression of Dichotomous and Seriousness Criteria on Offender and Environment Characteristics

Criterion type	Increment in R-sq.	F-test
Dichotomous (Success/failure)		
Predictor cluster		
Time available and offender characteristics	.224	$F(17,423) = 7.04$, $p < .001$
Environmental characteristics	.000	$F(1,422) = 0.20$, n.s.
Environment and offender interactions	.012	$F(5,417) = 1.33$, n.s.
Unmeasured environmental effects	.055	$F(1,416) = 32.49$, $p < .001$
Total R-sq. = .292; $F(24,416) = 7.14$; $p < .001$		
Seriousness score		
Predictor cluster		
Time available and offender characteristics	.246	$F(17,423) = 7.94$, $p < .001$
Environmental characteristics	.000	$F(1,422) = 0.19$, n.s.
Environment and offender interactions	.052	$F(5,417) = 6.17$, $p < .001$
Unmeasured environmental effects	.057	$F(1,416) = 36.17$, $p < .001$
Total R-sq. = .355; $F(24,416) = 9.55$, $p < .001$		

TABLE 8.2. Regression of Time Free and Seriousness/Time Free Criteria on Offender and Environment Characteristics

Criterion type	Increment in R-sq.	F-test
Time free		
Predictor cluster		
Time available and offender characteristics	.140	$F(17,264) = 2.42$, $p < .002$
Environmental characteristics	.000	$F(1,263) = 0.00$, n.s.
Environment and offender interactions	.071	$F(5,258) = 4.65$, $p < .001$
Unmeasured environmental effects	.043	$F(1,257) = 14.89$, $p < .001$
Total R-sq. = .255; $F(24,257) = 3.66$; $p < .001$		
Seriousness score/time free		
Predictor cluster		
Time available and offender characteristics	.066	$F(17,249) = 0.99$, n.s.
Environmental characteristics	.001	$F(1,248) = 0.30$, n.s.
Environment and offender interactions	.133	$F(5,243) = 8.05$, $p < .001$
Unmeasured environmental effects	.122	$F(1,242) = 43.51$, $p < .001$
Total R-sq. = .322; $F(24,242) = 4.79$, $p < .001$		

   Since our primary interest was in the environmental factor and its
interaction with offender characteristics, discussion of results relative to
time available and offender characteristics alone will be quite limited.
Time available is a significant predictor of three of the four outcomes
considered: the dichotomous measure (R^2 = .044; p < .001); the
seriousness measure (R^2 = .052; p < .001); and the time free measure (R^2
= .045; p < .001). Its contribution to the fourth criterion measure,
seriousness/time free, is not significant (R^2 = .002; n.s.).
   When considering the dichotomous criterion measure (which is similar
to those used in most prediction studies), offender characteristics
performed quite well, yielding results of substantially greater power than
typically has been observed (inclusion of offender characteristics resulted
in an increment in R^2 of .180). When combined with information
concerning time available in which to recidivate, the overall proportion
of variance in the dichotomous criterion accounted for was .224 (Table
8.1). Similar results were observed with respect to the seriousness criterion
(Table 8.1). When failures alone were considered, and the criterion was
either the length of time the offender remained free or the more complex
criterion which combined information concerning both time free and
seriousness, offender and time available characteristics performed
substantially less well (Table 8.2).

Socio-Environmental Characteristics

Considered net of time available to fail and offender characteristics, the
environmental scale proved not to be significantly associated with any of
the outcome measures studied (Tables 8.1 and 8.2). In other analyses, we
entered all socio-environmental variables available for study[15] into
regression equations controlling *only* for time available, and observed
increments in R^2 of less than 3% regardless of the outcome criterion
considered. In these equations, only the incivilities scale appeared to
have any consistent relation with the criterion measures.[16] In and of
themselves, then, it appears that the socio-environmental variables we
have explored here have little to do with release outcomes.

---

[15]These included the incivilities scale, the land-use scale, and three socio-
demographic variables from the only census data availability at the time
(proportion black population in 1980, 1970 average housing values, and 1970
average rental values).

[16]Hence our choice of that scale for inclusion in the analyses reported here.

Person-Environment Interactions

As we discussed, there are three general approaches one could take in attempting to predict recidivism: one could focus solely on characteristics of the offender (a trait or person approach); one could focus solely on the characteristics of the situation to which an offender is released (a situational approach); or one could focus on interactions between offender and environmental characteristics (an interactionist approach). In psychology (and in recidivism studies), the first two approaches have been pursued extensively. The trait approach has been criticized because validity coefficients for trait measures often are lower than .30 (Mischel, 1968; for an alternative view, see Hogan, DeSoto, & Solano, 1977). It is interesting to note that risk-screening devices also rarely (if ever) have coefficients larger than this (Gottfredson & Gottfredson, 1979). The influence of environments on behavior also has been well documented in psychology (Barker, 1968), and in addition to the ecological studies reviewed earlier in this chapter, has received attention in recidivism studies (Glaser, 1964; Monahan & Klassen, 1982; Reitzes, 1955).

Both in psychology (e.g., Wandersman & Florin, 1981) and in recidivism studies, we think that the interactionist approach holds promise. "Interactionism" has been used to refer to several different things (Buss, 1977; Olweus, 1977): in this study, our approach follows what Olweus called the "person-environment integrity" orientation. That is, we believe that the person, his/her environment, and his/her behavior interact in a process of mutual and reciprocal influence, and that these processes are an integral part of the environment. A first indication that this approach has validity would be the finding that different types of offenders perform differently in different types of environments.

Our basic hypothesis is confirmed: interaction terms do add to the predictive power of the regression equations, resulting in increments of 1% to 13% of the variance, depending upon the outcome criterion considered (Tables 8.1 and 8.2).

To aid in the interpretation of these interaction effects, we performed median-splits on each cluster of offender characteristics considered, and on the environmental incivilities scale. Typical interactions are displayed in Figures 8.1A and 8.1B, which graph interactions for the seriousness criterion considered. From examination of these figures, it is apparent that the nature and extent of the interactions depends not only on the outcome criterion considered, but on the particular class of offender attributes considered as well.

Figure 8.1A illustrates an interaction term based on offender risk assessed in terms of criminal history: prior arrests and incarcerations as a juvenile and as an adult. As the figure demonstrates, those offenders with an extensive history of criminal involvement ("bad risk" offenders) fail

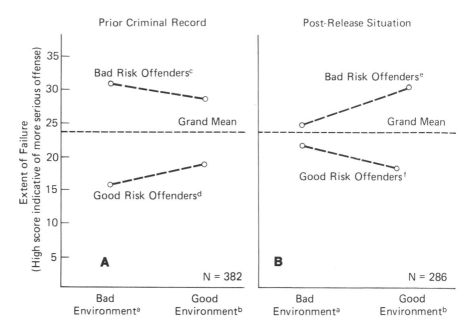

FIGURE 8.1. Interaction effects: seriousness criterion.
[a]Above median on Environmental Incivilities Scale.
[b]Below median on Environmental Incivilities Scale.
[c]Extensive prior record as juvenile and adult; based on median split.
[d]Moderate prior record as juvenile and adult; based on median split.
[e]Post-release situation assessed as poor at time of release in terms of financial need, vocational skills, employment status and stability, and wages; based on median split.
[f]Post-release situation assessed as good at time of release in terms of financial need, vocational skills, employment status and stability, and wages; based on median split.

more seriously when released to "bad" environments, and do better if released to "good" environments.[17] Note, however, that "good risk" offenders do *better* in poorer environments and more poorly in better ones. Such an observation is at variance with an "anomie" theory of criminality (Merton, 1957), which would anticipate that socially disorganized environments would have a deleterious effect on all released offenders. However, we observed no main effect for environment; instead, we observed this apparently counterintuitive interaction.

At this point it is important that we again stress the nature of our

---

[17]Our use of the terms "bad" and "good" environments should be considered simply as shorthand for neighborhoods whith high and low scores on the incivilities measure. No perjorative connotation is intended.

criterion measure, and the nature of the at-risk characteristics under consideration. For the analyses reported here, the outcome criteria were based on arrests only. At this stage in our research, conviction or incarceration criteria were problematic due to missing information. The at-risk characteristics considered in Figure 8.1—prior criminal involvement—were those which may well be related to surveillance by police and/or by members of the community. In "bad" environments, there not only may be more opportunities for failure, but there might also be considerably more formal (i.e., police-initiated) surveillance. Further, such surveillance might well be targeted on offenders with extensive criminal records. If so, reliance on surveillance by policing authorities could easily result in the pattern observed here: "good risk" offenders do better, and "poor risk" offenders more poorly, in socially disorganized environments. In better (more socially organized) environments, there may be less reliance on formal surveillance-control mechanisms, and an increased reliance on informal surveillance and control. Accordingly, "bad risk" offenders (perhaps not known to residents in the same way that they are known to police), do relatively better (they still do quite poorly, but in fact do better in better neighborhoods). "Good risk" offenders, on the other hand, do somewhat worse in the better neighborhoods. Although they may be "under-watched" by policing authorities, they may be watched by their neighbors. Thus, it would seem that a differential surveillance-control model—which results in a differential arrest/charging phenomenon—could be invoked to explain the observed interaction.

Figure 8.1B illustrates that the nature of the interaction can change dramatically when different offender risk-characteristics are considered. The figure graphs an interaction term based on an assessment of the offender's post-release situation (made at approximately the time of release). Considered in this scale are assessments of financial need and dependency, vocational skills, and employment status and stability. As the figure illustrates, offenders released to "bad" environments fail about equally seriously, but "good" environments have a deleterious effect on "bad risk" offenders, and a beneficial effect on "good risk" offenders. To us, these observations seem consistent with an opportunity model; and this seems particularly appealing given that the at-risk characteristics considered are economic ones, and that the effect is somewhat stronger for "bad risk" offenders. Not only may targets be more appealing in better neighborhoods, but agents of formal control may be less apparent— enhancing perceived opportunity. It also may be that a different sort of differential surveillance model is operating. In poorer environments, policing authorities may concentrate attention on offenders who are at risk due to prior criminal involvement (e.g., Figure 8.1). However, offenders who are at risk due to financial dependency and other economic considerations may be less salient in poorer environments, but considerably more salient—and particularly to neighbors—in better environments. Thus, we may be observing a differential surveillance effect, but here the effect may operate through informal, rather than formal, mechanisms.

Table 8.3 summarizes principal aspects of the interactions we have observed. As the table illustrates, the general nature of the interactions are consistent across different outcome criteria. For example, offenders at risk due to prior criminal involvement are more likely to be arrested in poorer neighborhoods and are free for shorter periods of time. They also have higher seriousness scores due to the fact that they are more likely to be arrested; however, when only failures are considered, the seriousness effect appears to be meliorated. To us, this seems very consonant with a differential surveillance hypothesis.

When we consider at-risk characteristics related to economic/financial dependency factors, an opportunity/need model seems more appropriate. Thus, poor risk offenders released to better neighborhoods (a) fail more frequently, and (b) fail more seriously, but (c) are free for longer periods of time.

Unmeasured Environmental Effects

A different approach to the examination of the effects of neighborhood or environment on release outcome focuses on neighborhood *per se*.[18] To this point, our discussion has focused on selected, measured aspects or characteristics of neighborhood environments which were deemed likely to have an impact on recidivism (although as we have stressed, most of the measures used were crude proxies for the concepts of interest). This approach will ask whether the neighborhood environment as a whole (but net of those characteristics which we already have assessed) has some impact on recidivism.

The general approach which we followed has been outlined by Bielby (1981) and Heise (1972). The inclusion of 66 dummy variables (since there are a total of 67 neighborhoods in the sample) in a regression equation is cumbersome and the equation quickly becomes unwieldy. Accordingly, we followed a two-stage model to develop a neighborhood variable or "sheaf coefficient" (Heise, 1972). Twelve neighborhoods contained but a single offender; these served as the reference group in a vector of dummy variables classifying the remaining 55 neighborhoods. These dummy variables were then regressed on recidivism. Resulting regression coefficients thus represented the adjusted mean difference in recidivism between each neighborhood and the reference neighborhoods. We then used these coefficients as one variable in a standard regression frame-

---

[18]We are indebted to Huey T. Chen for suggesting these analyses.

TABLE 8.3. Summary of Interaction Effects Across Outcome Criteria

| | Offender risk characteristics[a] | | | |
| | Criminal history risk | | Economic risk | |
	Good risk offenders	Bad risk offenders	Good risk offenders	Bad risk offenders
Environmental characteristics—"Good" environment (low incivilities)	More arrests in follow-up period Higher seriousness score Approximately same time-free as in 'bad' environments Offenders who fail do so more quickly/seriously	Fewer arrests in follow-up period Lower seriousness score Longer time-free Offenders who fail do so with approximately equal quickness/seriousness as in 'bad' environments	Fewer arrests in follow-up period Lower seriousness score Longer time-free Offenders who fail do so less quickly/seriously	More arrests in follow-up perior Higher seriousness score Longer time-free Offenders who fail do so more seriously/quickly
Environmental characteristics (high incivilities)	Fewer arrests in follow-up period Lower seriousness score Approximately same time-free as in 'good' environments Offenders who fail do so less quickly/seriously	More arrests in follow-up period Higher seriousness score Shorter time-free Offenders who fail do so with approximately equal quickness/seriousness as in 'good' environments	More arrests in follow-up period Higher seriousness score Shorter time-free Offenders who fail do so more quickly/seriously	Fewer arrests in follow-up period Lower seriousness score Shorter time-free Offenders who fail do so less quickly/seriously

[a]Comparisons made by column, *not* by row.

work assigning each neighborhood the regression coefficient for its dummy variable and repeating the earlier regression. This required use of only one additional variable (rather than sixty-six). Results are presented in Tables 8.1 and 8.2: inclusion of these unmeasured neighborhood effects on the final step resulted in increases in R^2 of from 4% to 12% over and above the increases provided by the measured neighborhood characteristics and their interactions with offender characteristics.

Of course, the interpretation of this finding is difficult since, by definition, we do not know to what to attriubte the effect (other than to neighborhood differences). It is interesting to note, however, that the contributions provided by the unmeasured characteristics follow the same general pattern as that provided by the interaction effects of the measured characteristics, becoming larger when more complex outcomes were considered.

Summary and Limitations

Results of these preliminary investigations are encouraging. As expected, we were able to increase predictive power through the inclusion of environmental characteristics. In general, these increases were principally due to interaction effects of environmental and offender characteristics. The observed effects were statistically significant and also appeared theoretically meaningful, particularly from an interactionist perspective. Person-environment interactions appeared most promising when criterion variables were more complex than simple success/fail dichotomies. Indeed, when very complex criteria were used, person-environment interaction effects exceeded main effects for offender characteristics in magnitude. Finally, it is clear that our relatively crude assessments have failed to capture fully the variation in neighborhood characteristics associated with criminal recidivism. Considerable environmental variation remains to be measured if we are to understand the nature of the observed person-environment interactions.

We must note some limitations to the research that we have presented here. First, we were unable (because 1980 census materials were substantially delayed in release to researchers) to assess adequately the effects of socio-economic and demographic variables on the relations observed and outlined above. We see the careful examination of these effects to be critical. Since the ecological literature suggests that the effects of socio-economic and demographic variables (considered on an areal basis) are likely to be substantial, and since these factors are known to covary with other environmental characteristics (such as those we assessed in this preliminary study), it is crucial that we attempt to examine the effects of environmental characteristics net of socio-demographic characteristics. The problem may be stated simply: socio-

economic and demographic characteristics are known to covary w
crime-related behaviors. Concepts such as social networks, cohesio
incivilities, and so on, are hypothesized to covary with crime-relate
behaviors, and appear to. Finally, social and demographic variables also
are known to covary with these concepts of social cohesion and incivility.
The research question is whether the concepts of cohesion, networks,
incivilities, and so on, are related to crime-related behaviors beyond their
relation to socio-economic and demographic characteristics.

Second, the environmental characteristics which we were able to
measure in this study were limited to observable physical characteristics.
It can be argued (and we argue strongly in the early part of this chapter)
that of the relevant neighborhood concepts, those measured here are less
likely to have predictive power than are others. Variables assessed here
stand only as crude proxies for things which one would prefer to measure
more directly, such as the nature and extent of local social networks,
social cohesion, and attachment.

Our current research efforts are devoted to overcoming both limitations.

Research Futures: An Interactionist Approach to Recidivism

On one level, the interactionist perspective is very simple: it is a statement
that behavior is a function both of the person and the environment; as
Lewin (1936) put it, $B = f(P,E)$. If we want to achieve an understanding of
how these influences function, however, definitions of interactionism
become more complex (Buss, 1977). Olweus (1977) has proposed four
different interactionist perspectives. He calls the first a *unidirectional*
perspective. Here, both person and environment variables are seen to
contribute to explanations of particular behavioral outcomes, although
no interplay between the person and environment predictors—in terms
of person variables being constrained (in their explanatory power) by
environment variables, or being potentiated by environmental variables—is assumed or predicted.

A second perspective is the *analysis of variance* approach. Here, it is
suggested that Person × Environment interaction terms (in an analysis of
variance framework) will contribute significantly to the explanation of
behavioral outcomes. The interaction terms may have more explanatory
power than either the Person or Environment main effects, although this
is not a necessary proposition of this perspective. The essential point is
that the person and environment variables bear a conditional relation to
each other.

A third perspective is the *reciprocal action* approach, which suggests
that the person and the environment influence each other reciprocally.

These influences result in adaptation and accommodation, such that changes in both the person and the environment result (i.e., the person and the environment transform each other over time). One assumption of this model would appear to be that a condition of congruence between the person and the environment evolves over time.

Olweus calls the fourth perspective on interactionism the *person-environment integrity* model. This approach suggests that the person, the environment, and the person's behavior in that environment are interwoven or integrated in a system-like fashion; that these three classes of variables have a functional integrity; and that this is reflected in processes of reciprocal influence. These different elements function as a single unit (similar to behavior settings; see Barker, 1968).

Statistically, our approach to interactionism looks like the fairly mechanistic analysis of variance approach, and this is correct. This study was limited both in scope and "depth" of information gathered, thereby restricting us to this mechanistic approach of testing for interactionism.

It should not be inferred, however, that we believe this mechanistic approach to be the appropriate conceptual framework for assessing community impacts on released offenders. Indeed, we feel that the person-environment integrity model will prove most useful. First, the offender's adjustment in the release environment represents not only the influence of the environment on the person, but the person's influence on that environment. The environment may influence the offender's behavior in many ways. By itself, it may serve as a discriminating stimulus to elicit some behaviors which are reinforcing, such as drug abuse. The environment produces social agents who may encourage either behaviors leading to recidivism, or behaviors leading to successful adjustment. Social agents may indirectly influence the course of events by encouraging police or other crime-control agents to keep track of the offender. Physical and land-use factors may be a source of influence by providing targets or opportunities for crime (or by limiting these). Thus, there are many ways in which the environment can have an influence on the released offender and the offender's behavior.

Likewise, there are many ways in which the offender and his/her behavior may influence the environment. The mere presence of an offender, if known to police or to community residents, may be a cause of increased vigilance, watchfulness, concern, or perhaps fear. Of course, the offender's behavior contributes to the environment by making it more or less orderly. If the offender's behavior becomes extremely antisocial, leading to the actual commission of crime(s), then this becomes an additional factor influencing environmental quality. Through his/her presence, then, as well as through his/her behavior, the offender may contribute to or detract from the quality of community life, and may stimulate local formal or informal control mechanisms.

Finally, we believe that offender behaviors leading to successful or unsuccessful adjustment are best (and most meaningfully) understood within the context of the release environment. Thus, the question of interest changes from "Did the offender get rearrested?" to "Where did this occur? Who was the victim (or where was the target)? Who were the accomplices? What encouragement was given by local peers? What was his/her employment situation at the time?" It is questions of this sort which ultimately must be addressed, and which ultimately will determine the extent to which we understand person-environment interactions in relation to recidivism.

Acknowledgments: Research reported here was supported by grants from the National Institute of Justice. Opinions expressed are solely those of the authors and do not necessarily reflect the official positions or policies of the United States Department of Justice. Huey T. Chen, Arnold J. Hopkins, and Sally A. Shumaker provided valuable assistance during the course of these investigations. Portions of earlier versions of this paper were presented at the meetings of the American Psychological Association (Anaheim, California, August 1983) and the American Society of Criminology Denver, Colorado, November 1983).

9
Firearms Ownership and Violent Crime: A Comparison of Illinois Counties

David J. Bordua

Introduction

As the title states, this is a study of firearms ownership and violent crime which is an extension of earlier work on firearms ownership in Illinois (Bordua & Lizotte, 1979; Bordua, Lizotte, & Kleck, 1979; Lizotte & Bordua, 1980; Lizotte, Bordua, & White 1981). However, the focus of this chapter is quite different in the following regard. In the earlier studies firearms ownership was the dependent variable. In this study violent crime rates are the dependent variables and the research explores the relationship of firearms ownership to violent crime.[1] The earlier research included both aggregate and individual-level analyses. The present study includes more detailed and weapon-specific data on violent crime as well as more sophisticated measures of the types and numbers of firearms owned.

Studies relating aggregate measures of firearms ownership to aggregate measures of violent crime have been rare—presumably because measures of ownership are difficult to construct. Survey data on ownership, now available nationally, are not available for comparison of states or smaller units of analyses. Aggregating survey data on the level of national regions results in aggregated units too large and internally heterogenous for useful analysis (Lizotte & O'Conner, 1979; Murray, 1975; Newton & Zimring, 1969). As was pointed out by Bordua and Lizotte (1979), the use

---

[1]Three subanalyses will be referred to as the analysis of General Ownership, Ownership Types, and Household Firearms. The first two are conducted at both bivariate and multivariate levels using the counties. The analysis of Household Firearms uses nine regions of the state.

The subanalyses use different measures of firearms ownership. The first, General Ownership, uses county rates of possession of Illinois Firearms Owners Identification Cards (FOIC). The second, Ownership Types, combines the FOIC rates and data from three statewide surveys. The third measures numbers of firearms in households using only the survey data.

of counties in Illinois has the advantage that the 102 counties are more homogenous than states and, since they are in the same state, share the same basic legal climate. Finally, the use of data from Illinois provides a unique opportunity to refine our measurement of firearm ownership because this state has a computerized file of Firearms Owners Identification Cards (FOIC) that can be the basis of county-level estimates of firearms ownership. Inclusion of firearms-ownership questions in three of the annual statewide surveys conducted by the Practicum in Survey Research of the Department of Sociology of the University of Illinois has resulted in the accumulation of considerable individual-level data as well.

Hypotheses and Causal Interpretation

Two recent books provide extensive reviews of the social science literature on firearms ownership and its possible relationships to violent crime (Wright, Rossi, & Daly, 1983; Kates, 1984). As a result, no systematic review of the literature will be attempted here.

The paucity of prior studies relating firearms to violent crime on an aggregate, cross-sectional basis makes the statement of detailed hypotheses difficult. The usual "commonsensical" expectation is that more guns or more owners means more crime. However, previous Illinois research indicates (e.g., Bordua & Lizotte, 1979; Lizotte, Bordua, & White, 1981) that the statistical relationships may not be positive. Individual-level results in the general literature and both individual and aggregate results in prior Illinois studies indicate moreover that even positive relationships may be causally ambiguous. If firearms ownership is positively related to aggregate crime rates in a cross-sectional analysis it may be that crime is causing an increase in gun ownership rather than the reverse. The general issue of causal interpretation is especially well discussed in Wright et al. (1983).

In this introductory section the issues will be stated and we will indicate where prior research has provided the basis for possible causal interpretations. In the last section of this chapter the causal inferences consistent with the empirical results will be presented. In dealing with the problem of causal ambiguity we can initially refer to three interrelated bodies of literature on firearms ownership: purposes for ownership; longitudinal studies of change in ownership and crime; and sex differences in ownership.

The survey literature on purposes for owning firearms is reviewed in detail by Kleck (1984). In nine studies conducted between 1975 and 1981, among those households or persons owning a firearm, anywhere from 28% to 73% (depending on the type of firearm) report protection as a primary or secondary reason for their ownership. The higher figure is from a survey on *individual* Illinois owners conducted by this author and colleagues. When those owning only a handgun or handguns were asked for their purposes, 73% gave protection as either the primary or secondary purpose (Bordua, Lizotte, & Kleck 1979: pp. 224, 231).

Studies of the relationship of fear of crime and/or actual crime rates or personal victimization to defensive ownership have produced mixed results. A careful review of this research, however, reveals that at least some of the studies suffer from serious deficiencies. In what Wright, Rossi, and Daly (1983) called the most sophisticated study to date the results were as follows. The county violent-crime rate positively affected respondents' perceived level of crime which positively affected fear of crime which in turn had a significant positive effect on gun ownership for protection. Additionally, personal victimization had a positive effect on fear which then affected protection ownership (Lizotte, Bordua, and White, 1981; see also Lizotte & Bordua, 1980). At the individual level then, there is credible evidence that sizeable proportions of owners own primarily or secondarily for protective reasons, and that protection ownership at least in Illinois is a consequence, at least in part, of variations in crime rates.

Among the longitudinal studies relating changes in firearms stocks to changes in violent crime, the best are those by Kleck which use national data and homicide as the dependent variable (Kleck, 1979; 1984). In the second and more sophisticated of the two studies the models are consistent with the interpretation that increases in homicide cause increases in the firearms stock but not the reverse except for an indirect positive effect through the robbery rate (Kleck, 1984: pp. 119–122).

Clotfelter (1981) in a study heavily criticized by Kleck concluded that the relationship of crime rates to handgun acquisition at the aggregate level was positive when no trend variable was included but non-significant when the trend variable was included. Clotfelter also concluded that national riots led to increased handgun acquisition. McDowell and Loftin (1983) in a time-series analysis of Detroit concluded that residents buy more handguns in response to violent crime and civil disorders.

The Kleck results would lead us to interpret a positive relationship between firearms ownership and violent crime as meaning that "crime causes guns" rather than the other way around. At the very least his results legitimate a conclusion that a positive relationship could mean either causal direction. It is not clear however whether the longitudinal results in Kleck are applicable to a cross-sectional analysis. Moreover, in a cross-sectional analysis there is no easy way to substitute for the lagged variable analysis Kleck was able to use.

We can go some way toward clearing things up by looking at sex differences in ownership. As has been stated, this chapter continues a series of studies on firearms ownership in Illinois by the author and colleagues. In that series special attention has been paid to sex differences in firearms ownership. In the earliest of the studies using Illinois counties, (Bordua & Lizotte, 1979) female ownership rates were predicted to be a positive function of county violent-crime rates while no prediction was made for males. The female ownership-crime relationship turned out to be curvillinear with a slightly negative relationship below the mean of county crime rates and a positive relationship above. The male ownership rate turned out to be negatively related to county violent-crime.

At the individual level (i.e., using survey data) female owners are much more likely to own handguns (as opposed to rifles and shotguns) than are male owners and are much more likely to give protection or defense-related reasons for ownership. At both the aggregate and individual levels then, we have reason to believe that female ownership would be *positively* related to violent crime rates and that the appropriate interpretation would be that the female ownership was a response to, rather than a cause of, crime.

Several other points can be made with respect to sex differences. Whether measured by FOIC holding or survey data, Illinois males are far more likely to own firearms than are Illinois females. In individual level models of firearms ownership for sport and protection this male predominance persisted. However, in a model of ownership for protection which included ownership for sport, sex proved nonsignificant, but in the direction of greater female ownership. This reinforces the point that females are much more likely to own for protection if they own (Lizotte, Bordua, & White, 1981:p. 501). If female ownership for protection is an especially important part of female ownership, we would expect that women who might have unusual protection needs would have unusual frequencies of firearms ownership for protection. In a survey of Illinois households in 1977, black females were 6.8% of the sample and 21.7% of those who owned purely for protection. The comparable figures for white women were 50.6% of the sample and 43.9% of the purely protection owners (Bordua, Lizotte, & Kleck, 1979:p. 218). Data such as these on the social distribution of protection ownership have implications not only for our analysis of firearms ownership and violent crime, but also obviously for firearms regulation policy (Bordua, 1983; 1984).

The Illinois studies also indicate that women's protection ownership may have been undergoing change. While purposes cannot be determined from FOIC data, two things can. Women are an increasing proportion of cardholders, having shifted from 4.6% of cardholders in 1970 to 8.1% in 1976 and 11.3% in 1984 (Bordua, 1985:p. 27). An earlier study found that between 1970 and 1976 male and female county ownership-rates showed a tendency to diverge (Bordua, Lizotte, & Kleck, 1979:p. 29). Linkage of women's ownership rates to traditionally male-dominated sport culture seemed to be giving way to more divergent patterns. If, as is plausible to suspect, this is an increase in women's protection ownership, then we can expect in the future to find a greater tendency for grossly measured firearms-ownership rates to be related to violent crime in causally ambiguous ways.

Thus the longitudinal analysis by Kleck indicates that a positive firearms-crime relationship *may* mean that crime causes firearms rather than the more "commonsensical" reverse. Individual-level data on purpose for owning and the relation of crime rates and personal victimization to protection ownership point in the same direction as does the data on female ownership.

Finally, we can look at weapon type. Crime with firearms is disproportionately with handguns. If we could estimate aggregate handgun-ownership rates separately and handgun ownership rates were positively related to violent crime, then it would be more plausible to argue that the higher firearms ownership was a cause of the higher violent crime rates. In fact, later in this chapter we test a more complex theory about handguns and crime. We hypothesize that the relationship of county rates of handgun ownership to violent crime will depend on the firearms "mix" or ownership type.

Ignoring the matter of weapons mix, the weapon-type hypothesis conflicts with the sex of owner hypothesis since, in Illinois at least, women owners are so disproportionately likely to be handgun owners. For causal interpretation purposes we can deal with the conflict, at least in part anyway, by appealing to known differences between the sexes in violent crime rates. Male violent crime rates are so much higher than the female rates that we can be skeptical that female ownership even of handguns will cause an increase in violent crime. A positive relationship between male handgun ownership and crime, however, would lend weight to the interpretation that the ownership was, at least in part, a cause of the crime.

Sporting Culture Effects

When asked the purpose of reason for firearms ownership, owners overwhelmingly give some sort of sporting- or hunting-related response. Indeed, hunting-license rates were used as proxy measures of firearms ownership in an early analysis comparing state crime rates (Krug, 1968). In their analysis of Illinois county ownership rates Bordua and Lizotte (1979) and Bordua, Lizotte, and Kleck (1979) demonstrated that male firearms ownership rates—as measured by FOIC holding rates—are positively related to such county-level indicators of sporting culture as hunting licenses and rates of subscription to the following sporting magazines: *Field and Stream*, *Outdoor Life*, and *Sports Afield*. These sporting-culture indicators were negatively related to a measure of county violent crime rates.

We would expect then, in the present analysis that at the zero-order level male firearms ownership would be negatively related to violent crime. It is plausible, however, that this negative relationship is in part produced by the effects of variations in sporting activity or "sporting culture." The sporting-culture variables are strongly correlated in the earlier research with situational and demographic variables which in turn predict violent crime. Since there are no obvious theoretical reasons for sporting culture as such to be predictive of violent crime, the model used in the multivariate analysis here includes only social and demographic variables. To a degree, controlling these variables also controls aggregate variations in ownership purposes or "cultures."

If the negative male ownership relationship persists, we can entertain provisionally the interpretation that male firearms ownership causes a *reduction* in violent crime. If the relationship is positive controlling the situational and demographic predictors, we can entertain the interpretation that net of the variables-controlled male ownership causes an *increase* in violent crime.

Male Ownership and Firearm Type

The sporting culture is largely, though by no means entirely, centered around long guns—rifles and shotguns. If we can estimate county ownership rates of different weapons, then we can make differential predictions about the direction of relationship and support different causal interpretations. In an earlier study using statewide telephone surveys done in 1976 and 1977, individual firearms owners were classified by what were called Ownership Types (Bordua, Lizotte, & Kleck, 1979). The types were defined in terms of the mix of firearms owned: Long Gun Only, Handgun and Long Gun, Handgun Only.

Given the previously cited data on sporting culture and ownership and weapon type and crime, we predicted that if a plausible causal interpretation is to be made among males where all three types are well represented, the relationship with violent crime rates would be negative for Long Gun Only, nothing or positive for Handgun and Long Gun, and Positive for Handgun Only. These would be predictions at the zero-order level. With multivariate controls for other social correlates of violent crime we would expect that if more firearms can plausibly be interpreted to mean more violent crime, then all relationships involving the male types might be positive or failing that, at least those involving Handgun Only and Long Gun and Handgun. In the analysis to follow we also combine the two handgun ownership types to test the effects of handgun ownership regardless of weapon mix.

Of course, positive relationships with male Handgun Only or any handgun ownership rates in a multivariate analysis still can leave causal direction, in principle, uncertain. Nevertheless if the type of potential offender (male) and the type of potential weapon (handgun) fit what is known about violent crime, then the case for positive causation is strengthened.

Theft, Passion, and General Availability

We have stated that if women's firearms ownership is positively related to county crime rate, it is plausible to interpret the relationship as a matter of crime causing gun ownership rather than the reverse. But such a relationship can be looked at rather differently. Regardless of the purpose for women—or anyone—owning, where there are more firearms there is a greater possibility of their coming (e.g., by theft) into the hands of people who might use them to commit crimes or indeed that they might turn an argument into an assault or murder even on the part of an owner originally motivated by protection.

This kind of general availability argument seems to underlie many of the recommendations of those who argue for stricter gun control as policy. For this argument to be plausible in our analysis it must be the case that male as well as female ownership be positively related to county violent crime rates. Moreover this "gun density" argument would be contradicted by any negative relationship between firearms ownership and violent crime produced by situational, demographic, or sporting-culture variables. If protection as an innocent purpose can lead to violent crime, then surely so can hunting or target shooting. While long guns are less often used in violent crime than are handguns, they certainly *can* be so used. Indeed, as has been recently argued with great force by Kleck (1984b), the superior "stopping power" of long guns makes them much more deadly than handguns and substitution of long guns for handguns at even a relatively modest fraction could increase rather than decrease serious injury and death.

The general availability or gun density argument is sometimes offered in terms of the crime of passion model—the ordinary citizen in a fit of rage seizes a firearm and kills without really "intending" to. This ordinary citizen model has come under serious criticism in general (Kleck & Bordua, 1984; Wright, Rossi, & Daly, 1983). For present purposes it would surely apply to long gun owners and pheasant hunters as much as to urbanites and handgun owners. The argument that handguns and passion somehow go together seems to mean either that sport firearms enthusiasts are devoid of passion or their weapons are inefficient. Paradoxically, since long guns and their owners are far more frequent than handguns and their owners, the "crime of passion-gun density" argument implies that the overwhelmingly most common form of ownership is relatively unlikely to produce crime—at least assaultive crime.

It seems implausible then to interpret any positive protection-oriented correlation with violent crime as an index of general availability of firearms and therefore a basis for an interpretation that guns cause crime rather than crime causing guns. In our data, for this to be true it would have to be the case that both male and female ownership would be positively associated and that both long gun and handgun ownership by either sex would be positively associated with crime.

Asymmetric Causal Interpretation

The analysis of firearms and crime does not stem originally from scientific but from rather selective reading of popular political and polemical concerns. In the parts of the popular debate attended to by social scientists, is almost entirely the potential for *increasing* crime that is discussed and the causal debate is largely conducted between those who argue that firearms ownership causes crime and those who say it does not. Only very small voices argue that firearms ownership may actually *reduce* violent crime; very small at least in the media to which sociologists are likely to be exposed. For an important exception to this rough generalization, however, see the recent paper by Blackman (1985).

As is so commonly the case, social scientists have taken over the causal debate largely intact from the political arena. Whether because they are relatively unexposed to pro-gun media, or because they have tended to sagecraft rather than science in the words of William Tonso (1984), it is only recently that they have entertained a more symmetrical view of causation. We need not go into great detail here, but the reader can be referred to discussions in Wright, Rossi, and Daly, (1983) and Kates (1984). This selective attention to directions of causality seems to have affected discussions of "defensible space"; space, it seems, to be defended by defenseless citizens. When the author once attempted to explain the theory of defensible space to a trapshooter friend, the friend pointed out that with a 12-gauge shotgun and double-ought buckshot his defensible space was at least 50 yards in every direction. He was assured that the theory meant something else.

If measures of firearms ownership are negatively related to violent crime, and if this relationship survives controls for the variables in the multivariate analysis, then we will have to entertain seriously the possibility that firearms ownership *reduces* violent crime.

Measurement

Illinois requires a Firearms Owners Identification Card (FOIC) before a firearm may be legally possessed. The FOIC system which has been in effect since July 1, 1968 is described in detail in a recent study (Bordua, 1985). The FOIC-based measures used here are from a special disidentified tape describing the valid cards as of mid-year 1976. The tape was provided by the then Illinois Department of Law Enforcement in 1976. Data on the cardholders is restricted to sex, age as of 1976, and county of residence. County rates of FOIC holding are the measure of firearms ownership in the first analysis of General Ownership. Since the FOIC system "registers owners, not guns" there are no data on types, patterns, or numbers of firearms owned or indeed on *owners* beyond the aforementioned.

The data on types of guns owned in the analysis of individual Ownership Types were secured from the statewide telephone surveys conducted in 1976, 1977, and 1981. For this analysis of types of ownership, an attempt is made to estimate county rates of three ownership types or patterns—Handgun Only, Handgun and Long Gun, and Long Gun Only. These individual ownership types are estimated using the survey data in combination with the FOIC county rates. Briefly, the combined total of owner cases in the three surveys was used to divide the state into regions. Within each region an estimate of the distribution of ownership types among owners was made and used as a weight for the FOIC rates of each of the counties in the region. Thus if a county with an FOIC rate of 20 per hundred was in a region where 25% of owners were Handgun Only, the county rate of Handgun Only ownership would be .25 (.20) = .05.

Three county-level Ownership Type rate estimates are derived by this procedure: one for all adults (18+), one for male adults, and one for female adults. The quality of the estimates varies in the same order. The estimates among adult owners are based on nine regions and 462 owners. The estimates for males are based on six regions and 375 owners. The female estimates are based on three regions and 87 owners.

The third analysis focuses on the number of firearms and the level of aggregation shifts from 102 counties to nine regions of the state. The regions are the same as those used for the overall ownership types. Household ownership of rifles, shotguns, and handguns is used as the base for the measure of firearms. Regional estimates of the number of firearms of each kind per 100 persons vary quite widely. In total guns per 100 the range is from 12.7 in Chicago to 76.7 in far West Central Illinois. In handguns per 100 persons the range is from 6.9 in East Central Illinois to 21.0 in North Central. Chicago is the second lowest on the list with an estimated 7.2 handguns per 100 persons.[2]

The 1976 Special FOIC Tape and the three statewide surveys enable development of a variety of county firearms ownership measures. As already stated in the introduction, the analysis of General Ownership is based purely on FOIC holding rates. The analysis of Ownership Types is

---

[2]In the correlational analysis reported in Table 9.6, Chicago is combined with the remainder of Cook County.

based on a mixture of FOIC rates and survey data on kinds of firearms owned. The analysis of Household Firearms in the nine Illinois regions uses ownership measures derived solely from survey data. The measures thus vary from more to less "contaminated" by legal compliance behavior—a point to be discussed after the results are presented.

The specific firearms-ownership measures used in the two subanalyses using counties are shown in the columns of Table 9.1. In the upper section are several purely FOIC-based measures. The top three in order are TOTALFOIC76—the county rate of ownership for all ages and both sexes; MALEFOIC76 and FEMALEFOIC76 are the sex-specific rates of card holding for adults 18 years and older. The next six measures in the upper section are age-specific rates of cardholding for males. These are included to assess the robustness of the findings.

The bottom three sections are devoted to the measures of Ownership Types. The first four measures are the Ownership Types with the sexes combined. The next four are for males and the bottom four are for females. In each of these sections the three Ownership Types are presented in the order Handgun Only, Handgun and Long Gun, and Long Gun Only. The last of each set of four measures combines Handgun Only with Handgun and Long Gun to give an overall estimate of the rates of ownership of handguns.

Before proceeding to a brief description of the violent crime measures, it is appropriate to introduce a caveat. Because the firearms measures vary in quality, the convention was adopted of emphasizing the general ownership measures first, the overall (combined sexes) ownership types second, the male types third, and the female types last. This is the order in which they are presented in the tables where they appear. If the general ownership measure showed no relationship, correlations involving the related ownership types should be treated with great suspicion—a rule to apply with special force to the female ownership types.

The data on violent crime were all secured from the Illinois Criminal Justice Information Authority (ICJIA). The first of the three series is labeled VIOLENT CRIME in Table 9.1 and has the Illinois UCR Index violent crimes of criminal homicide, forcible rape, robbery, and aggravated assault for the period 1972–80. The series also includes county data on simple battery—not used in Table 9.1. The second series is labelled WEAPON SPECIFIC and contains the I-UCR Index violent crimes by weapon *with the exception* of Index Criminal Homicide where weapons data were not available. Thus this data set is reported Index rape, robbery, and aggravated assault by weapon for the period 1972–81 *plus* Index criminal homicide without weapons data for the same period.

The third body of data called VICTIM LEVEL MURDER is a copy of a file created by ICJIA from the Supplementary Homicide Reports. The result is data on 10,585 murders in Illinois from 1973–81. Since weapons data were not available for all counties on I-UCR or UCR criminal homicide, this file is the source of information in analyzing county rates of criminal fatality by weapon. The file contains only data on murder and thus excludes nonnegligent manslaughter.

The 11 violent crime measures reported in Table 9.1 were selected to be of greatest theoretical interest but also with a stress on summary or total measures. The total measures are based on the largest numbers of reported violations and are presumably therefore more stable estimates.

In a study of firearms and violent crime, separate analysis of fatal crime has an obvious justification. The inclusion and exclusion of rape was done because earlier work on firearms in Illinois indicated that women's firearms ownership might be particularly responsive to violent crime rates. We attempted to see whether rape was of unusual significance. It was not.

The violent crime measures are the column headings in this table. Beginning on the left there are three measures from the VIOLENT CRIME file previously described. They are the TOTAL Illinois UCR reported Index violent crime offenses, NO RAPE (the TOTAL minus rape), and HOMICIDE (the I-UCR measure of reported criminal homicide). Measures in the middle panel are from the WEAPON SPECIFIC file for 1972–81. There are two summary measures of violent crime without firearms: NO FIREARM TOTAL of Aggravated assault, rape, and robbery is the Index violent crimes with firearms. NO FIREARM NO RAPE is just aggravated assault and robbery with firearms. The same conventions apply to the two measures FIREARMS TOTAL and FIREARM NO RAPE, these being obviously with firearms. In the WEAPON SPECIFIC segment the 1972–81 UCR criminal homicide measure is shown but not by weapon since that datum is not available for all Illinois counties. Finally, there are three measures of offenses known to the police from the VICTIM LEVEL MURDER file for 1973–81. The three measures there are self explanatory: VICTIM LEVEL MURDER TOTAL, NO FIREARM, and FIREARM are county rates for all murders, and murders without and with firearms respectively.

Bivariate Results: General Ownership

While it has become customary to skim lightly over bivariate results in modern quantitative sociology, the material in Table 9.1 deserves closer attention. This is believed to be the first body of data bearing with any serious precision on questions of aggregate firearms ownership and aggregate crime rates in a cross-sectional study. As a matter of convenience we can look at both the General Ownership and Ownership

TABLE 9.1. Bivariate Correlations Between County Rates of Firearms Ownership and County Rates of Violent Crime in Illinois[a]

Firearms ownership	Violent crime[b] 1972-80			Weapon specific[c] 1972-81					Victim level murder[d] 1973-81		
				No firearm		Firearm					
	Total	No Rape	Homicide	Total	No rape	Total	No rape	Homicide	Total	No Firearm	Firearm
General Ownership/FOIC											
TOTALFOIC76	-.48	-.48	-.24	-.44	-.43	-.43	-.43	-.21	-.29	-.31	-.23
MALEFOIC76	-.47	-.47	-.23	-.44	-.43	-.42	-.42	-.20	-.33	-.36	-.26
FEMALEFOIC76	.19	.19	.24	.17	.17	.25	.24	.25	.39	.15	.45
MALE18-24	-.49	-.48	-.26	-.47	-.46	-.46	-.46	-.23	-.39	-.34	-.35
MALE25-34	-.33	-.33	-.15	-.28	-.27	-.30	-.30	-.11	-.25	-.30	-.18
MALE35-44	-.43	-.43	-.21	-.39	-.38	-.37	-.37	-.18	-.27	-.33	-.19
MALE45-54	-.42	-.42	-.23	-.38	-.37	-.36	-.37	-.20	-.28	-.33	-.22
MALE55-64	-.38	-.38	-.21	-.36	-.36	-.30	-.30	-.18	-.24	-.30	-.17
MALE65+	-.32	-.32	-.13	-.27	-.26	-.27	-.27	-.12	-.13	-.22	-.06
Ownership Types/FOIC + Survey											
HANDGUNONLY	-.03	-.03	-.04	-.01	-.01	-.04	-.04	-.07	.02	-.02	.04
HAND&LONG	-.22	-.22	-.01	-.21	-.20	-.13	-.14	-.01	-.04	-.13	-.01
LONGUNONLY	-.42	-.42	-.26	-.39	-.38	-.41	-.41	-.22	-.32	-.28	-.29
HANDGUN	-.19	-.18	-.03	-.17	-.17	-.13	-.13	-.04	-.02	-.11	-.02
MALEHANDONLY	-.13	-.13	-.07	-.15	-.15	-.04	-.05	.06	.04	-.05	.07
MALEHAND&LONG	-.30	-.30	-.11	-.29	-.29	-.22	-.22	-.10	-.11	-.20	-.05
MALELONGONLY	-.38	-.38	-.26	-.34	-.33	-.40	-.40	-.22	-.38	-.33	-.34
MALEHANDGUN	-.26	-.26	-.05	-.26	-.25	-.17	-.17	-.05	-.07	-.16	-.01
FEMALEHANDONLY	.18	.18	.16	.16	.15	.17	.17	.18	.24	.17	.24
FEMALEHAND&LONG	.14	.14	.23	.13	.13	.24	.24	.22	.40	.13	.47
FEMALELONGONLY	.12	.12	.20	.13	.13	.19	.19	.20	.32	.07	.40
FEMALEHANDGUN	.23	.23	.27	.21	.20	.28	.28	.27	.44	.22	.47

[a] With N of 102, P < .05 when r = .17.
[b] Illinois Uniform Crime Reports violent crimes: Homicide, Rape, Aggravated Assault, Robbery. Prepared at author's request by Illinois Criminal Justice Authority (ICJIA).
[c] Illinois Uniform Crime Reports violent crimes by weapon—excludes homicide for which weapon data not available. Prepared at author's request by ICJIA.
[d] Based on Supplementary Homicide Reports. Victim Level Murder file created by ICJIA.

Type bivariate results and then shift in Table 9.2 to the multivariate results for these two subanalyses.[3]

General Ownership

The most general measure of firearms ownership rates for Illinois counties is in the top row of Table 9.1; TOTALFOIC76. The rate of Firearm Owners Identification Card holding in the 102 Illinois counties is negatively related to all the measures of violent crime in the table. These negative correlations are all statistically significant. Taking gun ownership in its most general sense and violent crime measured quite generally, more gun owners is related to less crime. In Table 9.1 this finding is true for crimes with and without guns and for measures with and without rape.

The overall negative relationship for general ownership does not persist when we look at the sex specific rates of cardholding in the second and third rows of Table 9.1. These are rates of cardholding by adults age 18 and over. The male adult ownership measure MALEFOIC76 correlates negatively with all the violent crime measures and with approximately the same magnitude as does the total ownership measure. This is not surprising since firearms ownership and cardholding are so overwhelmingly male—over 90% in 1976.

For fourth through ninth rows of the table show age-specific male FOIC rates for six age groups. We will not discuss these further except to point out that all the coefficients are negative and only five fail to meet the .05 significance level cut off of .17. Obviously the male negative relationship is quite robust at least as far as age is concerned. With age and sex being such prominent social correlates of violent crime, this pattern of findings among males is impressive.

With the row labeled FEMALEFOIC76 we see the obvious differences between the sexes. Comparing with male overall measures in the row above, we can see that *the male relationship is clearly negative and the female relationship is clearly positive.* The positive relationship of female ownership and crime is less strong than the negative relationship of male ownership except where the crime measure involves criminal fatality. For the two measures of I-UCR criminal homicide, the coefficients involving

[3]In interpreting the results shown in Table 9.1 there is great temptation to hunt for complex patterns and to overinterpret. This is aided by the fact that while it is discussed as a table of bivariate effects there are really four independent variables: ownership, sex, age, and ownership type along with 11 measures of violent crime. The coefficients are bivariate but the table overall is not. As far as possible, we will discuss main effects and overlook potential subtleties until the multivariate analysis.

males and females are approximately equal as is true for the total murder coefficients. With the exception of murder with a firearm, the lesser difference between the sex specific relationships is due to the fact that male negative coefficients are smaller rather than the female coefficients being clearly larger.

Conclusions: General Ownership

Several points can be made about the results thus far in the analysis of what we have called General Ownership. First, as measured most generally, (TOTALFOIC76) ownership of firearms is negatively related to violent crime. Second, this negative overall relationship is due to the negative relationship of male ownership. Third, the negative male ownership-violent crime relationship is quite robust as indicated by its universality in six male age groups. Fourth, female ownership is positively related to violent crime with the positive female coefficients being generally smaller than the negative male ones. Fifth, the differences in magnitude between the sex-specific coefficients do not seem to obtain for homicide and murder. This is mainly due to the fact that the male negative coefficients are smaller with these offenses. In the case of firearms homicide, the smaller male coefficient is paired with a much larger female ownership coefficient indicating that there may be some sex by offense interaction.

Causal interpretation is of course premature but at this point the only interpretations consistent with the earlier review would be that male ownership may be *reducing* crime and that crime may be *increasing* female ownership. Before further causal speculation it will help to look at the Ownership Types.

Bivariate Results: Ownership Types

In Table 9.1 the coefficients in the bottom three sections all involve measures of specific types of firearms and combinations of types. To review briefly, estimates of the county rates of ownership in the three types—Handgun Only, Handgun and Long Gun, and Long Gun Only— were developed by combining the county FOIC rates for 1976 with estimates of the distribution of types of firearms owned by owners derived from combining three statewide telephone surveys done in 1976, 1977, and 1981. The fourth measure in each section is an estimate of the county rate of ownership of handguns regardless of the other firearms types owned. As was done with General Ownership we will proceed by discussing the overall measures, that is, with the sexes combined first and then deal with the sex-specific relationships.

In the second panel of Table 9.1 where the Ownership Types for both

sexes are combined, two things seem apparent. First, there is a strong
Ownership Type effect. The rate of Long Gun Only ownership shows a
strong negative relationship to violent crime. Every coefficient in the row
headed LONGGUNONLY is negative and significant. Handgun Only
ownership shows no relationship. In the row headed HANDGUNONLY
the largest coefficient is −.07. The mixed Ownership Type in the row
headed HAND & LONG gives a mixed picture. All the coefficients are
negative but only four are significant. Second, at this level the theory
underlying the development of the ownership types seems only partially
supported. The shift is from clearly negative for Long Gun Only to very
uncertainly negative Handgun and Long Gun to no relationship at all for
Handgun Only.

The row headed HANDGUN, as we would expect from the results
above it, shows a rather uncertain pattern. There seems clearly no
relationship to the homicide and murder offenses with four significant
negative coefficients involving the other crime measures. Again the
verdict here should be something like "possibly weakly negative."

Sex of Owner and Ownership Types

As we would expect given the sex differences in general ownership and
the ownership-type effects just considered, the results in the bottom two
sections of Table 9.1 are rather complex. To begin with the males, the
Long Gun Only type of ownership is consistently negative and
statistically significant in its relationship to violent crime. Male Handgun
Only ownership is a bit more negative perhaps than was Handgun Only
in the previous panel but still basically nothing: eight of the coefficients
are negative but none are significant. The mixed pattern, Handgun and
Long Gun, shows clear negative relations with the violent crime measures
except for the measures of homicide and murder. The *order* predicted in
the theory underlying the ownership types is confirmed except that the
Handgun Only type is not positively related to violent crime.

Finally, among the males we can look at the coefficient in the row
headed MALEHANDGUN. Except for the homicide and murder
measures, they are fairly straightforwardly negative. Again we have an
indication that there may be some complex sex by weapon by offense
interactions. Certainly these male handgun ownership results do not
allow an interpretation that "the more handgun owners, the more crime."
Even with homicide and murder, the effects are nonexistent rather than
positive.

By comparison with the male ownership types, the females in the
bottom section give a picture of positive relationships. All 44 coefficients
in the section are *positive* in sign where 41 of 44 were negative in sign in
the male section. Thirteen of the female coefficients are not significant

statistically however. Beyond the general picture of positive coefficients the major finding of the bottom section is the bottom row, FEMALE-HANDGUN. Here all the coefficients are positive and significant. Dramatic evidence of the difference between the sexes can be found by comparing the female handgun row with MALEHANDGUN. Finally, in the lower right corner of the table we can see the persistence of the strong positive relationship between female firearms ownership and our measures from the Victim Level Murder file, particularly firearms murder.

Conclusions: Ownership Types

The theory underlying the development of what we called Ownership Types was only partially supported by the data in Table 9.1. We expected a negative relationship of Long Gun Only and crime, no relationship of Handgun and Long Gun, and a positive relationship of Handgun Only. Long Gun Only was indeed negative though only among males. Among males the mixed type, Handgun and Long Gun, was less negative in its relationship to violent crime and the Handgun Only type was essentially unrelated. Male handgun ownership disregarding type was negatively related to all eleven of the violent crime measures. Five coefficients were nonsignificant. All involved measures of homicide or murder.

As the Ownership Type conclusions thus far imply, there are important sex differences. The coefficients involving male ownership types are overwhelmingly negative. Those for female ownership are even more overwhelmingly positive. The female coefficients tend to be smaller and of the 44, 13 are not significant. The sex-specific analysis of ownership types, however, does not basically change the picture from the analysis of General Ownership—male negative, female positive. Female handgun ownership is especially clearly and positively related to violent crime rates. As another contrast with male Ownership Types the female relationships to the murder measures, especially firearms murder, are quite strong.

Despite the fairly dramatic sex and Ownership Type effects, the causal interpretations advanced earlier do not change much except to become more specific. The most clearly arguable interpretations are as follows: first, male long gun ownership *reduces* crime; second, crime *increases* female handgun ownership; third, *no* ownership pattern increases crime.

Less clearly arguable causal interpretations would be as follows: First, violent crime increases female ownership of all firearms types; second, except for purely long gun ownership, male ownership does *not* reduce homicide or murder; third, homicide and murder (especially firearms murder) increase female ownership unusually strongly.

Multivariate Results: The Firearms Variables in a Model of Violent Crime

In discussing the bivariate results, we made those causal interpretations that seemed most supportable by the relationships in Table 9.1. As was suggested in the introduction, however, causal interpretation is a logically difficult enterprise particularly in a cross-sectional study such as this. Whether it continues to be plausible to argue that male long gun ownership reduces crime and firearms murder increases female ownership, depends on whether either relationship survives being included in a multivariate model of county variations in violent crime rates. In addition, some relationships that are near zero in Table 9.1, such as male handgun ownership rates, may become positive in an appropriate model. So little multivariate research has been done relating firearms to violent crime that more sophisticated theorizing about likely outcomes is premature.

The earlier studies of firearms ownership in Illinois in general indicated that firearms ownership, particularly by males, tended to be rural while violent crime tended to be urban. It was also the case that firearms ownership tended to be high where there were few blacks while violent crime tended to be high where there were many.

As was mentioned in the introduction, one explanation of high rural ownership rates was the "sporting culture" centered around hunting. There is no plausible reason to expect "sporting culture" *per se* to be related either positively or negatively to violent crime, so sporting culture indicators were not included in the violent crime model used here.

The model of violent crime used in Table 9.2 was developed in studies of county rates of civilian firearms ownership in Illinois (Bordua & Lizotte, 1979). There a factorial measure of violent crime was used comprising rates of homicide, aggravated assault, and robbery. The exogenous variables that predicted the violent crime factor were: Percent Female-Based Households, 1970; Percent Urban, 1970; Population Density, 1970, and 18-34 Year-Old Blacks per capita, 1970. All relationships were positive. We call this model of social factors related to violent crime rates the Basic Model (i.e., without firearms measures).

For the multivariate analysis the age-specific male ownership measures were dropped leaving 15 firearms ownership measures. These combined with the 11 violent crime measures produce a total of 165 equations. Table 9.2 reports only the situations where the firearms ownership regression coefficient was significant at the .05 level. For these situations the sign of the coefficient is given along with the percent change in the adjusted R^2 produced by adding the firearms variable to the basic model. The adjusted R^2 for the basic model alone is given at the top of each column below the violent crime variable heading. Thus in the eleventh column headed **VICTIM LEVEL MURDER, FIREARM** the basic model produced an adjusted R^2 of .70318. Seventy percent of the variation in county rates of murder with a firearm is explained by the four variables of the basic model.

Of the 165 equations summarized in the table, 17 have firearms ownership coefficients meeting the statistical significance criterion. Of these, 13 are at the far right side of the table and involve the Victim Level Murder file. Within that group there are no significant coefficients involving nonfirearms murder.

Of particular importance is the fact that there are *no* significant coefficients where the data are from the Weapon Specific file and no significant coefficients involving either of the general measures of criminal homicide. To the left of the table there are four ownership-type coefficients, two each for male Long Gun Only and female Handgun Only. Since none of the measures of general ownership or the combined ownership type coefficients are significant, it seems appropriate to ignore these four.

Two findings leap out of the table. First, there is *no general relationship at all* between firearms ownership and violent crime rates comparing these Illinois counties. Generally speaking, *both* the negative male and positive female relationship disappear. Second, there *is* a positive relationship with firearms murder but not with criminal homicide generally.

Murder: Male Versus Female Ownership

The first finding of no general relationship is perhaps more practically significant. The second, relating ownership to firearms murder, is more intellectually mystifying. If we hark back to the material on causation presented earlier, we would have to argue that two causal interpretations are supported by the firearms-murder relationship. The positive relationship of male ownership to firearms murder rate should be most plausibly interpreted as ownership increasing crime. The positive relationship involving female ownership should be interpreted as supporting more the argument that this is a case of crime increasing firearms ownership.

These are not necessarily contradictory interpretations. It is quite possible to argue that the more males who own guns, the more firearms murder there is, and in turn the more females buy firearms for protection.

Such an interpretation is rendered suspect by some aspects of the findings in Table 9.1. The doubts center around the relationship of male ownership. Compared to the measures of female ownership, the picture with male ownership is rather weak. The addition to R^2 is lower for MALEFOIC76. Only one of the male ownership types is significantly related whereas all of the female ownership types are related to firearms

TABLE 9.2. Sign and Percent Addition to Adjusted R² Where Firearms Ownership Variable Significant in the Violent Crime Prediction Equation. (R² Without Firearms Below Crime Variable)

Firearms ownership	Violent crime 1972–80			Weapon specific 1972–81					Victim level murder 1973–81		
				No firearm		Firearm					
	Total .68512	No rape .68005	Homicide .32356	Total .57532	No rape .66229	Total .68332	No rape .68951	Homicide .27726	Total .68019	No Firearm .33935	Firearm .70318
TOTALFOIC76											+1.2%
MALEFOIC76											+2.2%
FEMALEFOIC76									+3.7%		+4.2%
HANDGUNONLY											
HAND&LONG											
LONGGUNONLY											
HANDGUN											
MALEHANDONLY	+1.6%										
MALEHAND&LONG											
MALELONGONLY		+1.5%									
MALEHANDGUN											+1.5%
FEMALEHANDONLY	+1.5%	+1.5%							+1.4%		+1.3%
FEMALEHAND&LONG									+1.4%		+2.0%
FEMALELONGONLY									+3.7%		+4.4%
FEMALEHANDGUN									+3.3%		+3.7%

murder and with sufficient strength to produce significant coefficients for the total murder rate. In short, we seem to have a weak male relationship and a strong female relationship.

Despite the preponderance of males among cardholders, none of the overall ownership types are related to murder or firearms murder. Finally, despite the preponderance of male offenders in studies of criminal homicide, there is no relationship of male ownership in Table 9.2 with the two measures of criminal homicide. In the Victim Level Murder file, for example, where sex of offender was known, only 14.8% were female. Where sex of offender and weapon were both known, only 11.5% of firearms offenders were female.

All of these considerations led to the hypothesis that the male ownership relation to firearms murder was spurious. Table 9.3 shows the pattern of interrelations among the firearms and murder measures at issue. As the table shows, it is possible that the positive correlation between MALEFOIC76 and FEMALEFOIC76 accounts for the weak positive relationship in the regression equation between male ownership and firearm murder.

The outcome of the statistical hypothesis would have implications for causal interpretation. If the male relationship proves spurious and the female persists, the most plausible interpretation will be that in the special case of firearms murder, variation in county crime rate is increasing firearms ownership rather than the reverse. If both persist, the most plausible interpretation was given earlier: the more male owners, the more firearms murder; the more firearms murder, the more female owners. Guns increase crime *and* crime increase guns. If the male relationship persists and the female disappears, then we must lean toward the interpretation that the gun ownership increases at least one kind of crime—firearms murder.

Putting the hypothesis of male ownership spuriousness to the test requires the use of the basic model plus the simultaneous use of male and female ownership measures. Table 9.4 and Table 9.5 show the tests of the hypothesis. In Table 9.4 the dependent variable is firearms murder and in Table 9.5 it is total murder—both from the Victim Level Murder file. In both tables a new firearms ownership measure is introduced labeled NOFEMFOIC76. This is TOTALFOIC76 minus FEMALEFOIC76— what is left of total FOIC-measured firearms ownership when adult female ownership is subtracted: adult male and subadult male and female ownership. This enables a test of whether the total ownership relation to firearms murder is due to the effect of female ownership.

Both tables show the basic model or equation to the left, add female adult ownership, and then add male ownership in the third equation. In the fourth equation the new measure with no adult female ownership is substituted for male ownership.

The key analysis is in Table 9.4. When both adult male and adult

TABLE 9.3. Correlations of Firearms and Crime Variables Involved in Tables 9.4 and Table 9.5

	TOTALFOIC76	MALEFOIC76	FEMALEFOIC76	NO ADULT FEMALE	TOTAL MURDER	FIREARM MURDER
TOTALFOIC76		.9620	.4756	.9715	-.2911	-.2328
MALEFOIC76			.3813	.9551	-.3277	-.3623
FEMALEFOIC76				.2534	.3930	.4492
NOADULTFEMALE					-.4261	-.3772
TOTALMURDER						.9494
FIREARM MURDER						

TABLE 9.4. Equations Predicting Illinois County Firearms Murder Rate per 10,000, 1973–81. Unstandardized Coefficients and Significance Levels Shown

Variable (sig.)	Basic equation	Female ownership	Female plus male	Female plus no adult female
% Fem. HH '70	.030601	.025712	.022897	.025635
	(.000)	(.002)	(.010)	(.003)
Pop/sq.mi. '70	.000032	.000053	.000056	.000053
	(.199)	(.030)	(.023)	(.031)
% Urban '70	.000280	.001117	.001381	.001129
	(.606)	(.053)	(.031)	(.095)
18–34 Blk. '70				
(per cap.)	12.764995	9.974546	11.176764	10.013160
	(0)	(.000)	(.000)	(.000)
FEMFOIC76		6.609664	5.486946	6.583504
		(.001)	(.016)	(.002)
MALEFOIC76			.263772	
			(.328)	
NOADULTFEM				.024307
				(.972)
Intercept	−.159625	−.298810	−.381850	−.301619
R	.84554	.86377	.86525	.86377
Adj. R²	.70318	.73288	.73279	.73077
F	60.81761	56.42065	47.16226	46.52828
Sig.	.000	.000	.000	.000

female ownership are included in the equation predicting firearms murder, male ownership drops out as a predictor while female ownership persists. The same happens to the new measures of ownership leaving out adult females. In Table 9.5 where the dependent variable is total murder, the results are the same. Female adult ownership persists, adult male and NOFEMFOIC76 do not.

Statistically adult female firearms ownership accounts for the effects of adult male ownership and overall ownership.

Causally only one plausible interpretation survives the analysis. At least one kind of crime increases at least one kind of firearms ownership. Firearms murder increases adult female ownership.

Conclusions: Multivariate Analysis

Tables 9.2-9.5 add up to the general finding that firearms ownership has no relationship to violent crime except that female ownership has a positive relationship to firearms murder and thereby to the total murder rate. The most plausible causal interpretation is that in the single case of firearms murder and female owners, violent crime increases gun ownership.

Table 9.5. Equations Predicting Illinois County Murder Rates per 10,000, 1973–81. Unstandardized Coefficients and Significance Levels Shown

Variable (sig.)	Basic equation	Female ownership	Female plus male	Female plus no adult female
% Fem. HH '70	.035136	.029054	.029564	.030894
	(.004)	(.013)	(.017)	(.011)
Pop/sq.mi. '70	.000092	.000185	.000118	.000117
	(.008)	(.001)	(.001)	(.001)
% Urban '70	.000620	.001661	.001613	.001368
	(.412)	(.040)	(.073)	(.148)
18–34 Blk. '70 (Per cap.)	15.478926	12.006921	11.789187	11.090489
	(0)	(.000)	(.000)	(.001)
FEMFOIC76		8.224045	8.427381	8.844883
		(.003)	(.009)	(.003)
MALEFOIC76			−.047772	
			(.900)	
NOADULTFEM				−.576884
				(.549)
Intercept	−.135440	−.308620	−.293581	−.241948
R	.83238	.84843	.84846	.84906
Adj. R^2	.68019	.70525	.70219	.70327
F	54.70419	49.33152	40.69085	40.89662
Sig.	.000	0	.000	.000

Household Firearms

The third empirical analysis uses nine Illinois regions rather than the 102 Illinois counties—the same regions used to derive the overall Ownership Types. The firearms data are from the three statewide surveys in 1976, 1977, and 1981. Combined, the three surveys provided 2267 cases—too few to use county level units; thus, the intrastate region level of aggregation. As has already been stated in the section on measurement, the survey interviews produced data on the household ownership of handguns, rifles, and shotguns. The average number of each kind of firearm owned in region households was multiplied by the number of households in the region to estimate the total number of each kind of firearm. This estimate is the numerator in the measures of firearms per hundred persons used in Table 9.6.

This third analysis contributes to the larger study in several ways. First, it counts guns rather than merely owners. Second, the firearms measures are purely survey in nature thus reducing problems of contamination by legal compliance involved in using the FOIC measures. Third, the level of aggregation is different though each region is a grouping of counties. Fourth, this is truly a measure of "gun density," a methodological point that will come up later.

Regional variation in the number of firearms per hundred persons is

TABLE 9.6. Estimated Firearms Per Hundred Persons and Violent Crime Rates in Nine Illinois Regions. (Entries Are Correlation Coefficients)

| Guns/100 persons | Violent crime 1972–80 | | | Weapon specific 1972–81 | | | | Victim level murder 1973–81 | |
	Total	No rape	Homicide	Total no Firearm	Total Firearm	Homicide		Total	Firearm
All guns	-.6995*	-.7051*	-.3711	-.7303*	-.5896*	-.3271		-.6421*	-.6076*
Handguns	-.3524	-.3505	-.4135	-.3113	-.3536	-.3998		-.3493	-.3327
Rifles	-.6641*	-.6693*	-.2765	-.6594*	-.5805*	-.2235		-.6689*	-.6438*
Shotguns	-.7527*	-.7619*	-.3247	-.8416**	-.5825*	-.2800		-.6359*	-.5899*

*P < .05
**P < .01

considerable. The estimated number for Chicago is 12.7. For deep Southern Illinois the estimate is 71.1. The highest estimate is for an area of West Central Illinois that largely comprises the "land between the rivers" (i.e., that part of the state lying between the Illinois and Mississippi rivers). Here the three combined surveys estimate that there are 76.8 firearms for each hundred persons. In the analysis reported in Table 9.6, Chicago is combined with the remainder of Cook County to constitute one of the nine regions.

With only nine regions within a single state it is not possible to do much in the way of creative analysis. The purpose here is mainly to provide a rough check on the results of the other two analyses. If the results of the regional analysis do not obviously contradict those of the earlier bivariate analysis using counties, then the credibility of the earlier results is greatly enhanced. This is especially the case because of the fact that firearms measurement is purely survey in nature.

Table 9.6 presents an abbreviated version of Table of 9.1 with firearms per hundred persons substituting for ownership measures, regions substituting for counties, and three of the crime measures omitted. They were excluded because the earlier analyses indicated that continuing the distinctions involving rape and nonfirearms murder would not be fruitful.

Four findings seem apparent in Table 9.6. First, measuring firearms rather than ownership does not seem to change the basically negative relationship of nonsex specific firearms measures to measures of violent crime. Second, coefficients involving the handguns per hundred variable while negative like the others are much smaller and in no case reach statistical significance: a result similar to the HANDGUN row in Table 9.1. The most important finding is that measuring the presence of firearms by purely survey methods produces results quite in agreement with those of the earlier analysis using Firearms Owners Identification Cards thus strengthening study findings against the potential criticism that the ownership measures partly measure aggregate tendencies to legal compliance (i.e., to legally register ownership). Finally, Table 9.6 indicates that here also the measures of firearms seem to be less negatively related to measures of criminal homicide.

Some Considerations of Measurement

Problems in measurement have been discussed at various points in this chapter. Were there in existence many cross-sectional aggregate studies relating firearms ownership to violent crime rates, a full fledged discussion would have had to appear in the beginning of this one. However, when nearly everyone is using axes, there is less need to explain Bowie knives.

Any method of measuring firearms ownership contains error. Hopefully, random but systematic error can have obvious effects on results of a study such as this. The most likely source of systematic error lies in the contamination of the ownership measures with aspects of "law-abidingness" or more broadly "social compliance" or conventionality. In order to be called a gun owner a subject must do something other than simply own a gun. In this study he or she must do one or both of two things—get an FOI card or answer telephone interview questions. In the first case, law abiding behavior; in the second, an exhibition of a degree of conventional accessability and willingness to participate in the interview. If these propensities toward law abidingness or "conventionality" are nonrandomly related to the crime rates of county or regional units used in this chapter, then problems could occur. It is an obvious hypothesis that the nonlaw abidingness and unconventionality displayed in violent crime might be correlated with these behavioral elements of our gun ownership measures. If so, we would expect that firearms ownership would be *underestimated* in the high-violence counties.

Our measures vary. The purely FOIC-based measures require an overt act of legal compliance. The ownership types are based mainly on the FOIC system and partly on survey interviews. The surveys require accessibility to and participation in interviews—a less "contaminated" measure than purely FOIC, presumably. At least a considerable number of the survey respondents in 1976 and 1977 were willing to admit having a gun but not having a card. The measures of household ownership require only the "conventional" behavior involved in being survey interviewed.

Thus, on a continuum from FOIC to ownership types to household ownership the measures are less potentially biased by "social compliance." Unfortunately the least-biased purely survey measues are available only for the coarse regions reported.

Movement from legal compliance (FOIC) to mixed legal and customary (Ownership Types) to purely customary (Household Firearms) does in fact increase the number of persons reporting firearms ownership. For the combined 1976 and 1977 surveys 72% of owners reported that they *did* have FOI cards. Analysis of the self-admitted noncarded owners indicates that female owners are more likely to be noncarded than are male owners—49% to 24%. In an earlier study considerable analysis was done of regional distribution of noncarded owners within the state. To quote the earlier report:

Based on these data at least, and again other than women firearms owners, we did not discover any concentration of owners *without* cards except in social locations where there were concentrations of owners with cards. (Bordua, Lizotte, & Kleck, 1979; p. 172)

Obviously this does not settle the measurement problem. It does indicate however that measurement requiring less legal and/or customary compliance might produce quite unexpected results (e.g., a large increase in women owners but little or no geographical change). It should also be pointed out that the only going alternative method of measuring firearms presence for small social units is the so-called "gun density" measure. This uses the percentage of homicides and suicides performed with firearms as a measure of the prevalence of firearms. If some of our measures are contaminated by legal compliance and social convention-ality surely this measure is contaminated by a tendency to use firearms in violent acts.

Using such a measure, Cook (1979) studied the relationship of "gun denisty" to robbery, firearms robbery, and robbery murder. The findings in part agree and disagree with those of this study. Gun density in a multivariate model of 50 cities had no relationship to the overall robbery rate but a positive relationship to the firearms robbery rate and to the rate of robbery murder. Cook concluded that while guns did not make robbery more common they seemed to make it more dangerous. Cook validated his measure of gun density by correlating city "gun-density" measures with regional firearms ownership as measured by surveys.

The Cook study made no attempt to measure ownership by sex or to deal with the complex issues of causal interpretation that have been raised here. As one analyst has pointed out, the positive relationship could at least in part be a matter of gun robbery and robbery murder producing gun ownership (Kleck, 1984:103). No one knows whether this causal reversal is in fact true, however, and understanding the differences between Cook's measures and findings and these in Illinois will require considerable further work. The fact that our intrastate regional analysis involving a true "gun-density" measure based solely on survey data gives negative relations justifies skepticism about the Cook findings but no more.

One possible interpretation of Cook's positive findings involves his use of the 50 largest cities. It may be that large cities are "crime prone" and variation in firearms prevalence may mean something quite different than it would in our sample of counties. Moreover, there is nothing in Cook's sample corresponding to the sporting-culture context of firearms ownership mentioned in the introduction. The meanings of firearms ownership may differ greatly. Ownership of guns for sport may mean that they are owned by neither the dangerous nor the endangered.

This of course introduces the larger subject of interaction effects. Our research shows basically that variations in firearms ownership do not increase violent crime. There may, however, be social contexts where more gun owners does mean more crime—another topic for future research.

As one final measurement comment, it should be pointed out that the combination of measures used here, whatever their weakness, is clearly more adequate than others in the literature for cross-sectional research. Moreover, a quite considerable variation is measured on the firearms variables. As has been pointed out, within Illinois regional numbers of firearms per hundred persons varies from 12.7 to 76.8. The percentage of households owning any kind of firearm varies from 18.9 to 59.8. At the county level the percentage of the population with an FOI card varies from 6.8 to 23.7. Among adult males the percentage range is 20.5 to 59.4.

It is possible that any positive effect on violent crime would take place only below these lower values. This would imply some exceedingly complex nonlinear relationships between firearms ownership and violent crime if we had areas with ownership levels more nearly zero. It would also imply that policies to reduce violent crime by reducing firearms ownership would have to reduce ownership by extremely large fractions to have any effect.

Deadliness and Percentage Use of Firearms

The analysis of firearms ownership and crime in Illinois which we set out to do is completed. Findings, conclusions, and causal interpretations appear in the text and will be briefly summarized in the next section.

The basic conclusion that firearms ownership variation has *no* relationship to violent crime follows from the use of crime rates as dependent variables. It is of special interest that the nonrelationship obtains for homicide and, excepting women's ownership, for murder. It is also of special interest that where we had weapon-specific rates there is no relationship between firearms ownership and crimes with firearms—again excepting female ownership and firearms murder.

We would expect firearms to be more likely positively related to homicide because the effect can be two-pronged. Guns might increase the rate of attacks *and* guns might make attacks more deadly (Kleck & Bordua, 1984). We might also conjecture that firearms may make people more violent but that they may not use the guns in the attacks; in which case we would find a positive correlation between firearms ownership and attacks without firearms. This is essentially the argument put forward in the famous pop psych argument that the trigger may be pulling the finger (Berkowitz, 1968). The experimental literature on the subject has been reviewed extensively by Kleck and Bordua (1983, 1984.) They conclude that experimental findings " . . . suggest that, for the population as a whole, guns are as likely to *inhibit* assaults as to incite them, and that gun ownership therefore has no effect at all on the frequency of assaults" (p. 31).

Attacks with firearms are by definition aggravated assault/battery and would be included in our dependent variables. Assaults without firearms

TABLE 9.7. Firearms Ownership Rates of Illinois Counties Related to Nonfirearms Attacks, Firearms Attacks, Deadliness and Percentage Use of Firearms

Firearms ownership	(1) Simple battery[a]	Aggravated assault[b]		(4) Deadliness[c]	% Use of firearms	
		(2) No firearms	(3) firearms		(5) Total. w/o murder[d]	(6) Tot. with murder[e]
General Ownership/FOIC						
TOTALFOIC76	-.53	-.40	-.41	.03	-.21	-.19
MALEFOIC76	-.51	-.40	-.40	.02	-.18	-.16
FEMALEFOIC76	-.03	.18	.25	.04	-.07	-.05
MALE18-24	-.48	-.44	-.45	-.03	-.20	-.19
MALE25-34	-.37	-.25	-.29	.02	-.18	-.16
MALE35-44	-.47	-.35	-.35	.05	-.08	-.05
MALE45-54	-.44	-.34	-.34	.00	-.18	-.17
MALE55-64	-.42	-.33	-.28	.01	-.06	-.04
MALE65+	-.44	-.23	-.25	.05	-.19	-.18

Ownership Types/FOIC+Survey						
HANDGUNONLY	−.09	−.00	−.07	−.04	−.11	−.11
HAND&LONG	−.33	−.19	−.13	.13	.02	.03
LONGGUNONLY	−.40	−.36	−.38	−.03	−.22	−.21
HANDGUN	−.30	−.15	−.14	.09	−.03	−.02
MALEHANDONLY	−.29	−.15	−.08	.12	−.01	−.00
MALEHAND&LONG	−.41	−.26	−.21	.09	−.03	−.02
MALELONGONLY	−.31	−.30	−.37	−.08	−.21	−.20
MALEHANDGUN	−.39	−.24	−.18	.10	−.03	−.02
FEMALEHANDONLY	.14	.13	.15	−.04	−.13	−.11
FEMALEHAND&LONG	−.12	.14	.24	.11	.05	.06
FEMALELONGONLY	−.11	.15	.23	.04	−.06	−.04
FEMALEHANDGUN	.03	.19	.27	.04	−.07	−.05

[a] Violent Crime File, Simple Battery, 1972–80.
[b] Weapon Specific File. Aggravated Assault/Battery, 1972–81.
[c] Deadliness calculated from Violent Crime File, 1972–80. Index is: $\dfrac{\text{Homicide}}{\text{Homicide+Aggravated Assault}}$
[d] Weapon Specific File, 1972–80. Percent of Rape, Robbery and Aggravated Assault commited with a firearm.
[e] Weapon Specific File, 1972–81. Victim Level Murder File, 1973–81. Percent of Rape, Robbery, Aggravated Assault (1972–81) plus Murder (1973–81) committed with a firearm.

may or may not be aggravated and included. Simple battery by definition in Illinois cannot include *any* deadly weapon. It may also be the case that attacks with firearms are differentially reported to the police thus biasing empirical relationships.

As a final point, firearms may not make aggravated assaults more likely or more deadly and may not make homicide/murder more likely. Firearms may also not make people more attack prone even without weapons. It may be that firearms do not produce any higher probability of violence at all but do increase the likelihood that where violence occurs the percentage with firearms will be higher.

Table 9.7 shows data bearing on all these points. It is useful to compare the results with those in Table 9.1. The first two columns, Simple Battery and Aggravated Assault Without Firearms, show that overall ownership and male ownership are negatively related to both measures of attacks without firearms. At this level at least firearms ownership does not instigate nonfirearms attacks. The point is most clear when considering Simple Battery.

The third column of Table 9.7 looks quite similar to the second. Aggravated assault with firearms relates essentially the same way to firearms ownership as does aggravated assault without firearms.

The fourth column shows the results of an aggregate county-level measure of deadliness. The Index of Deadliness uses data from the Violent Crime file for 1972-1980. It is the ratio for each county of homicide to homicide plus aggravated assault. The idea for such an index comes from a publication by Zimring (1968) in which he develops a similar index to compare firearms and nonfirearms assaults. Kleck (1984) develops a much more elaborate indicator of relative deadliness in comparing the deadliness of assaults with long guns and handguns for use in assessing possible consequences of a control policy that led to substitution of the former for the latter. In Table 9.7 there is no relationship of any of the firearms ownership measures to this crude measure of deadliness. It does not seem to be the case that gun ownership either makes attacks more frequent and more deadly or less frequent and more deadly.

The final point—the percentage contribution of reported crimes with firearms to the total of reported crimes—is addressed in the right-hand columns in Table 9.7. These columns use data from the Weapon Specific file for 1972 to 1981 and the Victim Level Murder file for 1973 to 1981. Column 5 is the county percentage of all reported violent crimes committed with firearms *excluding* homicide or murder. In column 6 the dependent variable includes murders from the Victim Level Murder file. Since some counties had no murders, percentage use of firearms in murder could not be analyzed separately.

Columns 5 and 6 show some persistence of negative relations with overall and male ownership and a persistence of the negative relationship with Long Gun Only ownership by males.

The findings in Table 9.7 are bivariate and perhaps would not survive sophisticated multivariate controls. No attempt was made to construct models for these dependent variables because existing theory does not specify appropriate variables other than the firearms-ownership variables and these are already in the analyses. We should also point out that the lack of relationship between our firearms-ownership measures and the measures of percentage use reinforces the point that further research is needed on the differences between our measures of ownership and the "gun density" measure used by Cook (1979).

Summary and Conclusions

The statistical findings of the study are easy to summarize. In the bivariate analysis of General Ownership and violent crime using Illinois counties, overall ownership was negatively related to violent crime. When sex-specific General Ownership was investigated, male ownership continued to be negative while female was positive. The negative male-ownership relationship persisted when six age groups of male owners were distinguished.

In the bivariate study of Ownership Types we predicted that Long Gun Only would be negatively related to crime, Handgun and Long Gun would be unrelated, and Handgun Only would be positively related. The predictions were only partially supported. Long Gun Only ownership is indeed negatively related to violent crime though only among males. Indeed, this seems largely though not entirely to account for the negative relationship of male general ownership. Among males the mixed type, Handgun and Long Gun, was less negative than Long Gun Only and the Handgun Only ownership was essentially unrelated. There are important sex differences in the Ownership Type results. The coefficients involving male ownership types are overwhelmingly negative. Those for female ownership, though smaller, are even more overwhelmingly positive.

In the multivariate analysis of General Ownership and Ownership Types the overarching finding is that both male negative and female positive results were wiped out when the firearms ownership variables were used in a model of county variations in violent crime derived from earlier research in Illinois. The exception was murder and firearms murder from the Victim Level Murder file. Total overall ownership and both male and female ownership were positively related to firearms murder rates. For a number of reasons it was hypothesized that female ownership would account for the relationships involving total and male ownership. The hypothesis turned out to be true.

As far as statistical findings are concerned we are left with only the findings that murder and firearms murder rates are positively related to female firearms ownership comparing Illinois counties. An analysis of nine Illinois regions where crime rates were related to a measure of firearms per hundred persons was generally supportive of the county level results. Empirical analysis ended in Table 9.7 with a series of specialized inquiries tangential to the main inquiry. At the bivariate level ownership is related to rates of nonfirearms attack the same way as to firearms attack. It does not produce a tendency toward attacks without firearms—the trigger does not pull the finger. Firearms ownership does not make attacks more deadly at least at this aggregate level. Finally, there is no relationship between our ownership measures and the percentage use of firearms in violent crime.

Causal interpretations do not flow automatically from statistical results, especially the results of cross-sectional analyses. Early in the text the plausibility of various causal interpretations was discussed and the reasoning will not be repeated here. The most plausible interpretation resulting from the study is that variation in firearms ownership has no independent causal affect on violent crime at all. A less important though analytically interesting interpretation is that murder, especially firearms murder, has a positive causal effect on women's firearms ownership.

Issues of causal interpretation do not end here however. It is conceivable that the "no relationship" in the multivariate model is due to counterbalancing effects. If we knew more about who owned firearms, it would be possible to test the hypothesis that ownership by some segments of the population *reduces* crime while high crime rates *increase* ownership among other segments, thus producing no relationship. At the present time, however, this hypothesis remains untested; and as such, it represents another avenue for future research on firearms and crime.

Acknowledgments: A revision and expansion of a paper read at the 1984 Annual Meetings of the American Society of Criminology in Cincinnati, Ohio. The research reported here was supported by a grant from the Research Board of the University of Illinois at Urbana-Champaign. Mark Beeman served as Research Assistant and his contribution is gratefully acknowledged. The measures of violent crime used were provided by the Illinois Criminal Justice Authority; J. David Coldren, Director. Staff members who were especially helpful were Carolyn Rebecca Block and Louise S. Miller, Senior Research Analysts and former staff member Lawrence Dykstra. Finally the assistance of Joe L. Spaeth, Director of the Practicum in Survey Research, University of Illinois at Urbana-Champaign is much appreciated.

References

Akers, R. L. (1980). Further critical thoughts on Marxist criminology: comments on Turk, Toby, and Klockars, pp. 133–138 in J. A. Inciardi (Ed.), *Radical criminology: The coming crises*. Beverly Hills: Sage.

Allison, P. D. (1977). Testing for interaction in multiple regression. *American Journal of Sociology 83*, 144–153.

Avio, K. L. & Clark, C. S. (1976). *Property crime in Canada: An econometric study*. Published for the Ontario Economic Council by the University of Toronto Press.

Bailey, W. (1984). Poverty, inequality, and city homicide rates: Some not so unexpected findings. *Criminology 22*, 531–550.

Baldwin, J. (1979). Ecological and areal studies in Great Britain and the United States, pp. 29–66 in N. Morris & M. Tonry (Eds.) *Crime and justice: An annual review of research*. Chicago: University of Chicago Press.

Baldwin, J. (1975). British areal studies in crime: An assessment. *British Journal of Criminology 15(3)*, 211–227.

Baldwin, J. (1974). Social area analysis and studies of delinquency. *Social Science Research 3*, 151–168.

Baldwin, T. & Bottoms, A. E. (1976). *The urban criminal: A study in Sheffield*. London: Tavistock Publications.

Ball-Rokeach, S. J. (1973). Values and violence: A test of the subculture of violence thesis. *American Sociological Review 38(6)*, 736–749.

Bane, M. (1985). Household composition and poverty: Which comes first? Paper presented at the conference on "Poverty and Policy: Retrospect and Prospects," Williamsburg, Virginia.

Banfield, E. C. (1970). *The unheavenly city*. Boston: Little, Brown.

Barker, R. (1968). *Ecological Psychology*. Stanford, CA: Stanford University Press.

Bates, W. (1962). Caste, class and vandalism. *Social Problems 9*, 349–358.

Beasley, R. W. & Antunes, G. (1974). The etiology of urban crime: An ecological analysis. *Criminology II, 4 (February)*, 439–461.

Belsley, D., Kuh, E., & Welsh, R. (1980). *Regression diagnostics*. New York: John Wiley.

Berecochea, J. E., Himelson, A. M., & Miller, D. F. (1972). The risk of failure during the early parole period: A methodological note. *Journal of Criminal Law, Criminology, and Police Science 63*, 93–97.

Berkowitz, L. (1968). Impulse, aggression and the gun, *Psychology Today* *2(September)*, 22.

Berry, B. J. L. [Ed.] (1972). *City classification handbook: Methods and applications.* New York: Wiley Interscience.

Berry, B. J. L. & Kasarda, J. D. (1977). Contemporary urban ecology. New York: Macmillan.

Bielby, W. T. (1981). Neighborhood effects: a LISREL model for clustered samples. *Sociological Methods and Research 10*, 82–111.

Blackman, P. H. (1985). Carrying handguns for personal protection: Issues of research and public policy. Presented at the annual meeting in November of the American Society of Criminology. San Diego.

Blalock, H. (1982). Conceptualization and measurement in the social sciences. Beverly Hills, CA: Sage.

Blau, J. R. & Blau, P. M. (1982). The cost of inequality: Metropolitan structure and violent crime. *American Sociological Review 47(1)*, 114–129.

Block, R. (1977). *Violent crime: Environment, interaction and death.* Lexington, MA: Lexington Books.

Block, R. (1975). Homicide in Chicago: A nine year study (1965–1973). *Journal of Criminal Law and Criminology 66 (December)*: 496–510.

Block, R. & Zimring, F. (1973). Homicide in Chicago 1965–1970. *Journal of Research in Crime and Delinquency 10 (January)*, 1–12.

Blumstein, A. & Larson, R. C. (1971). Problems in modeling and measuring recidivism. *Journal of Research in Crime and Delinquency 8*, 124–132.

Booth, A., Johnson, D., & Choldin, H. (1977). Correlates of city crime rates: Victimization surveys versus official statistics. *Social Problems 25*, 187–197.

Bordua, D. J. (1985). Operation and effects of firearms owners identification and waiting period regulation in Illinois. (Mimeo. X + 189 pp.)

Bordua, D. J. (1984). Gun control and opinion measurement: Adversary polling and the construction of social meaning. In D. B. Kates, Jr., (Ed.), *Firearms and Violence: Issues of public policy.* Pacific Institute for Public Policy Research. Cambridge, MA: Ballinger Publishing Company.

Bordua, D. J. (1983). Adversary polling and the construction of social meaning: Implications in gun control elections in Massachusetts and California. *Law and Policy Quarterly 5 (July)*, 345–366.

Bordua, D. J. (1958–1959). Juvenile delinquency and anomie: An attempt at replication. *Social Problems 6*, 230–238.

Bordua, D. J. & Lizotte, A. J. (1979). Patterns of legal firearms ownership: A cultural and situational analysis of Illinois counties. *Law and Policy Quarterly 2 (April)*, 147–175.

Bordua, D. J., Lizotte, A. J., & Kleck, G. with Van Cagle (1979). Patterns of firearms ownership, use and regulation in Illinois. (A report to the Illinois Law Enforcement Commission. Mimeo, XVIII + 253 pp.).

Braithwaite, J. (1979). *Inequality, crime and public policy.* London: Routledge and Kegan Paul.

Brantingham, P. & Brantingham, P. [Eds.] (1981). *Environmental criminology.* Beverly Hills: Sage Publications.

Brantingham, P. & Brantingham. P. (1984). *Patterns in crime.* New York: MacMillan.

Burgess, E. W. (1925). Can neighborhood work have a scientific basis? pp. 142–

155 in R. E. Park, E. W. Burgess, & R. McKenzie (Eds.), *The City*. Chicago: University of Chicago Press.

Bursik, R. J., Jr. (1984). Urban dynamics and ecological studies of delinquency. *Social Forces 63*:

Bursik, R. J., Jr., & Webb, J. (1982). Community change and patterns of delinquency. *American Journal of Sociology 88*, 24–43.

Buss, A. R. (1977). The trait-situation controversy and the concept of interaction. *Personality and Social Psychology Bulletin 3*, 196–201.

Byrne, J. (1984). Social ecology and criminal justice policy: The impact of ecological factors on decision making in the criminal justice system. (Paper presented at the annual meeting of the American Society of Criminology, Cincinnati, Ohio.)

Byrne, J. M. (1983). The ecological correlates of property crime in the United States: a macroenvironmental analysis. Ph.D. dissertation. New Brunswick: Rutgers University.

Campbell, T. H. & Bendick, Jr., M. (1977). *Public assistance data book*. Washington, DC: The Urban Institute.

Carroll, L. & Jackson, P. (1983). Inequality, opportunity, and crime rates in central cities. *Criminology 21*, 178–194.

Chaiken, J. M. & Chaiken, M. R. (1983). Crime rates and the active criminal, pp. 11–30 in J. Q. Wilson (Ed.), *Crime and Public Policy*. San Francisco, CA: Institute for Public Service Press.

Chilton, R. J. (1983). Age, gender, race and changes in urban arrest rates. Paper presented at the annual meeting of the American Sociological Association, Detroit.

Chilton, R. J. (1964). Continuity in delinquency area research: A comparison of studies for Baltimore, Detroit, and Indianapolis. *American Sociological Review 28 (1)*, 71–83.

Chilton, R. J. & Dussich, J. P. J. (1974). Methodological issues in delinquency research: Some alternative analyses of geographically distributed data. *Social Forces 53*, 73–82.

Chilton, R. J. & Spielberger, A. (1971). Is delinquency increasing? Age structure and the crime rate. *Social Forces 49 (March)*, 488–93.

Chilton, R. J. & Sutton, G. (in press). Classification by race and Spanish origin in the 1980 census and its impact on white and non-white races. *The American Statistician*.

Clark, J. & Wenniger, E. (1962). Socioeconomic class and area as correlates of illegal behavior among juveniles. *American Sociological Review 28*, 826–834.

Clotfelter, C. T. (1981). Crime, disorders and the demand for handguns: An empirical analysis. *Law and Policy Quarterly 3*, 425–446.

Cloward, R. A. & Ohlin, L. E. (1960). *Delinquency and opportunity*. New York: Free Press.

Cloward, R. A. & Piven, F. P. (1975). *The politics of turmoil: Poverty, race and the urban crisis*. New York: Vintage.

Cohen, J. & Cohen, P. (1975). Applied multiple regression/correlation analysis for the behavioral science. Hillsdale, NJ: Erlbaum.

Cohen, L. E. (1981). Modeling crime trends: A criminal opportunity perspective. *Journal of Research in Crime and Delinquency 18, 1 (January)*, 138–164.

Cohen, L. E. & Felson, M. (1979). Social change and crime rate trends: A routine activities approach. *American Sociological Reveiw 44*, 588–607.

Cohen, L. E., Kleugel, J., & Land, K. (1981). Social inequality and predatory criminal victimization: An exposition and test of a formal theory. *American Sociological Review 46*, 505–524.

Cook, P. J. (1981). The effect of gun availability on violent crime patterns. *Annals of the American Academy of Political and Social Sciences 455 (May)*, 63–79.

Cook, P. J. (1979). The effect of gun availability on robbery and robbery murder: A cross-section study of 50 cities. In R. Haveman & B. B. Zellner, (Eds.), *Policy studies review annual* Vol. III, pp. 743–81. Beverly Hills CA: Sage Publications.

Cook, P. (1983). The influence of gun availability on violent crime patterns, pp. 49–90 in M. Tomry and N. Morris (Eds.) *Crime and Justice (Volume 4)*. Chicago: University of Chicago Press.

Cook, P. (1975). The correctional carrot: Better jobs for parolees. *Policy Analysis 1*, 11–54.

Cooley, F. H. (1902). *Human nature and the social order*. New York: Scribners.

Coombs, C. H. (1967). Thurstone's measurement of social values revisited forty years later. *Journal of Personality and Social Psychology 6*, 91–92.

Coser, L. A. (1967). *Continuities in the study of social conflict*. New York: Free Press.

Council on Municipal Performance (1973). City crime: Report of the Council on municipal performance." *Criminal Law Bulletin 9 (7)*, 557–611.

Crenson, M. A. (1983). *Neighborhood politics*. Cambridge, MA: Harvard University Press.

Cronbach, L. J. (1960). *Essentials of psychological testing*. New York: Harper.

Crutchfield, R., Geerken, M., & Gove, W. (1982). Crime rates and social integration: The impact of metropolitan mobility. *Criminology 20*, 467–478.

Cureton, E. G. (1967). Validity, reliability, and baloney, pp. 372–373 in D. Jackson and S. Messick (Eds.) *Problems in human assessment*. New York: McGraw-Hill.

Curtis, L. A. (1975). *Violence, race, and culture*. Lexington, MA: D. C. Heath.

Dahir, J. (1947). *The neighborhood unit plan: Its spread and acceptance*. New York: Russell Sage Foundation.

Danziger, S. (1976). Explaining urban crime rates. *Criminology 14, 2*, 291–296.

Danziger, S. & Wheeler, D. (1975). The economics of crime: Punishment or income redistribution? *Review of Social Economy 33 (2)*, 113–131.

Datesman, S. K. & Scarpitti, F. R. (1980). Female delinquency and broken homes: A reassessment, pp. 129–149 in S. Datesman & F. Scarpitti (Eds.) *Women, crime, and justice*. New York: Oxford.

Davidson, M. & Toporek, J. (1983). General univariate and multivariate analysis of variance and covariance, including repeated measures, in W. Dixon (Ed.) *BMDP Statistical Software*. Berkeley, CA: University of California Press.

Davies, M. (1969). *Probationers in their social environment*. London: Her Majesty's Stationery Office.

Dawes, R. W. (1979). The robust beauty of improper linear models in decision making. *American Psychologist 34*, 571–582.

Dawes, R. W. (1977). Case-by-case vs. rule-generated procedures for the allocation of scarce resources, pp. 83–94 in M. F. Kaplan & S. Schwartz (Eds.) *Human judgment and decision processes in applied settings*. New York: Academic Press.

Dawes, R. M. & Corrigan, B. (1974). Linear models in decision making. *Psychological Bulletin 81*, 95-106.

Decker, D., Shichor, D., & O'Brien, R. (1982). *Urban structure and victimization.* Lexington, MA: D. C. Heath.

Decker, S. H. (1977). Official crime rates and victim surveys: An empirical comparison. *Journal of Criminal Justice 5*, 47-54.

De Fronzo, J. (1983) Economic assistance to impoverished Americans. *Criminology 21 (1)*, 119-136.

Dentler, R. A. & Monroe, L. J. (1961). Social correlates of early adolescent theft. *American Sociological Review 26*, 733-743.

Duncan, O. D. & Schnore, L. F. (1959). Cultural, behavioral and ecological perspectives in the study of social organization. *American Journal of Sociology 65*, 132-145.

Dunn, C. S. (1980). Crime area research, in D. Georges-Abeyie and K. Harries (Eds.), *Crime: A spatial perspective.* New York: Columbia University Press.

Dunn, C. S. (1974). The analysis of environmental attribute/crime incident characteristic interrelationships. Ph.D. dissertation. Albany: State University of New York.

Einhorn, H. & Schact, S. (1980). Decisions based on fallible clinical judgment, pp. 126-144 in M. F. Kaplan & S. Schwartz (Eds.), *Human judgment and decision processes in applied settings.* New York: Academic Press.

Elliot, D. S., Agerton, S. S., & Canter, R. J. (1979). An integrated theoretical perspective on delinquent behavior. *Journal of Research in Crime and Delinquency (January)*: 3-21.

Erikson, K. T. (1966). *Wayward Puritans: A study in the sociology of Deviance.* New York: Wiley.

Erlanger, H. S. (1976). Is there a 'subculture of violence' in the South? *Journal of Criminal Law and Criminology 66*, 483-490.

Erlanger, H. S. (1974). The empirical status of the subculture of violence thesis. *Social Problems 22 (2)*, 280-292.

Faris, R. E. L. & Dunham, W. (1939). *Mental disorders in urban areas.* Chicago: University of Chicago Press.

Farrar, D. & Glauber, R. (1967). *Multicollinearity in regression analysis. Review of Economics and Statistics 49*, 92-107.

Federal Bureau of Investigation (1971). *Uniform crime reports—1970.* Washington, DC: U.S. Government Printing Office.

Felson, M. & L. Cohen. (1980). Human ecology and crime: A routine activity approach. *Human Ecology 8*, 389-406.

Ferdinand, T. (1970). Demographic shifts in criminality: An inquiry. *British Journal of Criminology 10 (April)*, 169-75.

Finestone, H. (1976). The delinquent and society: The Shaw and McKay tradition, pp. 23-49 in J. F. Short (Ed.) *Delinquency, crime, and society.* Chicago: University of Chicago Press.

Fischer, C. S. (1981). The public and private worlds of city life. *American Sociological Review 46 (June)*, 306-316.

Fischer, C. S. (1975). *Toward a subcultural theory of urbanism. American Journal of Sociology 80 (6)*, 1319-1341.

Fischer, C. S., Jackson, R. M., Steuve, C. A., Gerson, K., & Jones, L. M. (1977). *Networks and places: Social relations in the Urban Setting.* New York: Free Press.

Flango, V. E. & Sherbenou, E. L. (1976). Poverty, urbanization, and crime. *Criminology 14, 3 (November)*, 331–346.

Frederickson, G. [Ed.] (1972). *Neighborhood control in the 1970's* Lexington, MA: D. C. Heath.

Freed, D. & Wald, P. (1964). Bail in the United States: 1964. Working paper. National Conference on Bail and Criminal Justice (May).

Froland, C. & Pancoast, D. S. [Eds.] (1979). *Networks for helping: Illustrations from research and practice*. Portland, OR: Regional Research Institute, Portland State University.

Gans, H. (1968). *People and plans: Essays on urban problems and solutions*. New York: Basic Books, Inc.

Gans, H. (1962). *The urban villagers*. New York: The Free Press.

Garofalo, J. & Hindelang, M. (1977). An introduction to the National Crime Survey. Washington, DC: U.S. Government Printing Office.

Gastil, R. D. (1971). Homicide and a regional culture of violence. *American Sociological Review 36*, 412–427.

Georges-Abeyie, D. E. & Harries, K. D. [Eds.] (1980). Crime: A *spatial perspective*. New York: Columbia University Press.

Gerson, K., Steuve, C. A., & Fischer, C. (1977). Attachment to place, pp. 139–162 in C. Fischer et al. (Eds.) *Networks and places: Social relations in the urban setting*. New York: Free Press.

Gibbons, D. C. & Jones, J. F. (1975). *The study of deviance*. Englewood Cliffs, NJ: Prentice-Hall.

Gibbs, J. (1978). *Crimes against persons in urban, suburban, and rural areas: A comparative analysis of victimization rates*. Washington, DC: U.S. Government Printing Office.

Gibbs, J. J. (1978). A comparative analysis of household victimization rates in urban, suburban, and rural areas. (Analytic Report, Criminal Justice Research Center, Albany, New York.)

Gibbs, J. P. & Erickson, M. L. (1976). Crime rates of American cities in an ecological context. *American Journal of Sociology 82 (3)*, 605–620.

Gilder, G. (1981). *Wealth and poverty*. New York: Bantam.

Glaser, D. (1964). *The effectiveness of a prison and parole system*. New York: Bobbs-Merrill.

Glenn, N. D. (1967). Massification versus differentiation: Some trend data from national surveys. *Social Forces 46 (December)*, 172–180.

Glueck, S. & E. Glueck (1950). *Unraveling juvenile delinquency*. New York: Commonwealth Fund.

Goldkamp, J. (in press). *Policy guidelines for bail: An experiment in court reform*. Philadelphia: Temple University Press.

Goldkamp, J. (1979). *Two classes of accused: A study of bail and detention in American justice*. Cambridge, MA: Ballinger.

Goldkamp, J. & Gottfredson, M. R. (1979). Bail decision making and pretrial release: Surfacing judicial policy. *Law and Human Behavior 3 (4)*, 227–249.

Goodman, A. C. & Taylor, R. B. (1983). *The Baltimore neighborhood fact book: 1970 and 1980*. Baltimore, MD: Center for Metropolitan Planning and Research, The Johns Hopkins University.

Gordon, R. A. (1967). Issues in the ecological study of delinquency. *American Sociological Reveiw 32 (6)*, 927–944.

Gorsuch, R. L. (1974). *Factor analysis*. Philadelphia: Saunders.

Gottfredson, D. M. (1967). Assessment and prediction methods in crime and delinquency, pp. 171–187 in *Task force report: Juvenile delinquency and youth crime*. Washington, DC: U.S. Government Printing Office.

Gottfredson, D. M. & Ballard, K. B. (1964). Association analysis, predictive attribute analysis, and parole behavior. Paper presented at the meetings of the Western Psychological Association, Portland, Oregon.

Gottfredson, D. M. & Gottfredson, M. R. (1980). Data for criminal justice evaluations: some resources and pitfalls, pp. 97–118 in M. Klien & K. Teilman (Eds.) *Handbook of criminal justice evaluation*. Beverly Hills, CA: Sage.

Gottfredson, D. M., Wilkins, L. T., Hoffman, P. B., & Singer, S. M. (1974). *The utilization of experience in parole decision making: Summary report*. Washington, DC: U.S. Government Printing Office.

Gottfredson, M. R. (1974). An empirical analysis of pre-trial release decisions. *Journal of Criminal Justice 2*, 287–303.

Gottfredson, S. D. & Gottfredson, D. M. Screeening for risk among parolees: policy, practice, and method, pp. 54–77 in D. Farrington and R. Tarling (Eds.) *Prediction in Criminology*. Albany, NY: SUNY Albany Press.

Gottfredson, S. D. (1980). *Exploring the dimensions of judged offense seriousness*. Baltimore, MD: Center for Metropolitan Planning and Research, The Johns Hopkins University.

Gottfredson, S. D. (1980). Screening for risk. *Criminal Justice and Behavior 7 (3)*, 315–330.

Gottfredson, S. D. & Gottfredson, D. M. (1979). Screening for risk: A comparison of methods. Washington, DC: National Institute of Corrections.

Gottfredson, S. D. & Taylor, R. B. (1982). Person-environment interactions in the prediction of recidivism. Baltimore, MD: Center for Metropolitan Planning and Research, The Johns Hopkins University.

Gottfredson, S. D. & Taylor, R. B. (1983). *The correctional crisis: Prison populations and public policy*. Washington, DC: National Institute of Justice.

Gough, H. C. (1962). Clinical versus statistical prediction in psychology, pp. 526–584 in L. Postman (Ed.) *Psychology in the making*. New York: Knopf.

Granovetter, M. S. (1974). *Getting a job*. Cambridge, MA: Harvard University Press.

Granovetter, M. S. (1973). The strength of weak ties. *American Journal of Sociology 78*, 1360–1380.

Green, E. (1970). Race, social status, and criminal arrest. *American Sociological Review 35*, 476–490.

Greenberg, D. (1985). Age, crime, and social explanation. *American Journal of Sociology 91*, 1–21.

Greenberg, D. F. (1979). Delinquency and the age structure of society. *Contemporary Crises 1 (Apr.)*, 189–223.

Greenberg, S. W., Rohe, W. M., & Williams, J. R. (1984c). *Informal citizen action and crime prevention at the neighborhood level: Volume I*. Synthesis and assessment of the research. Report submitted to the National Institute of Justice. Research Triangle Park, NC: Research Triangle Institute.

Greenberg, S. W., Rohe, W. M., & Williams, J. R. (1984b). *Informal citizen action and crime prevention at the neighborhood level: Volume II.* Secondary analysis of the relationship between responses to crime and informal social control. Report submitted to the National Institute of Justice. Research Triangle Park, NC: Research Triangle Institute.

Gurr, T. R. (1970). *Why men rebel.* Princeton: Princeton University Press.

Hackney, S. (1969). Southern violence, pp. 505–528 in H. D. Graham & T. R. Gurr (Eds.) *History of violence in America. Report of the Task Force on Historical and Comparative Perspectives to the National Commission on the Causes and Prevention of Violence.* New York: Bantam.

Hakim, S. & Rengert, G. (1981). *Crime spillover.* Beverly Hills, CA: Sage Publications.

Harries, K. D. (1980). *Crime and the environment.* Springfield, IL: Charles C Thomas.

Harries, K. D. (1976). Cities and crime: A geographic model. *Criminology 14, 3 (November)*, 369–386.

Harries, K. D. (1974). *The geography of crime and justice.* New York: McGraw-Hill.

Harris, M. (1981). *America now.* New York: Simon and Schuster.

Hauser, D. & Schnore, L. F. [Eds.] (1965). *The study of urbanization.* New York: John Wiley and Sons, Inc.

Hawley, A. (1971). *Urban society: An ecological approach.* New York: The Ronald Press.

Hawley, A. (1950). *Human ecology.* New York: The Ronald Press.

Heise, D. R. (1975). *Causal analysis.* New York: Wiley-Interscience.

Heise, D. R. (1972). Employing nominal variables, induced variables and block variables in path analysis. *Sociological Methods and Research 1*, 147–173.

Henig, J. R. (1980). Gentrification and displacement within cities: A comparative analysis. *Social Science Quarterly 61*, 638–652.

Henry, A. F. & Short, Jr. J. F. (1954). *Suicide and homicide.* New York: Free Press.

Hindelang, M. (1981). Variations in sex-race-age-specific incidence rates of offending. *American Sociological Reveiw 46 (August)*, 461–74.

Hindelang, M. (1974). The uniform crime reports revisited. *Journal of Criminal Justice 2*, 1–17.

Hindelang, M., Gottfredson & Garofalo, J. (1978). *Victims of personal crime.* Cambridge, MA: Ballinger.

Hindelang, M., Hirschi, T., & Weiss, J. G. (1981). Measuring delinquency. Beverly Hills, CA: Sage.

Hindelang, M. J. (1978). Race and involvement in common law personal crimes. *American Sociological Review 43*, 93–109.

Hirschi, T. (1983). Crime and the family, in J. Q. Wilson (Ed.), *Crime and public policy.* San Francisco, CA: Institute for Contemporary Studies.

Hirschi, T. (1979). Separate and unequal is better. *Journal of Research in Crime and Delinquency (January)*, 34–38.

Hirschi, T. (1969). *Causes of delinquency.* Berkeley, CA: University of California Press.

Hirschi, T., & Gottfredson, M. (1985). Age and the explanation of crime. *American Journal of Sociology 89 (November)*, 552–84.

Hirschi, T., & Selvin, H. C. (1967). *Delinquency research: An appraisal of analytic methods.* New York: Free Press.

Hoch, I. (1974). Factor in urban crime. *Journal of Urban Economics 1*, 184–229.

Hoffman, P. B. & Beck, J. (1974). Parole decision-making; A salient factor score. *Journal of Criminal Justice 2, (3)*, 195–206.

Hogan, R., DeSoto, C. B., & Solano, C. (1977). Traits, tests, and personality research. *American Psychologist 33*, 255–269.

Holmes, W. (1981). ILK conditioning. Unpublished paper presented in workshop at Northeastern University, Center for Applied Social Research (March).

Holmes, W. (1979). Examining reliability and multicollinearity of scale items. *Behavioral Research Methods and Instrumentation 11*, 86.

Hunter, A. (1978). Symbols of incivility: Social disorder and fear of crime in urban neighborhoods. Paper presented at the meetings of the American Society of Criminology, Dallas, Texas.

Hunter, A. (1974). *Symbolic communities: The persistence of change in Chicago's local communities.* Chicago: University of Chicago Press.

Isaacs, R. R. (1948). The neighborhood theory: An analysis of its adequacy. *Journal of the American Institute of Planners 14*, 15–23.

Iversen, G. & Norpoth, H. (1976). *Analysis of variance.* Beverly Hills, CA: Sage.

Jacobs, D. (1981). Inequality and economic crime. *Sociology and Social Research 66*, 12–28.

Johnstone, J. (1978). Social class, social area and delinquency. *Journal of Sociology and Social Research 63*, 49–72.

Kasarda, J. & M. Janowitz. (1974). Community attachment in mass society. *American Sociological Reveiw 47*, 427–433.

Katzman, M. T. (1980). The contribution of crime of urban decline. *Urban Studies 17*, 277–286.

Keller, S. (1968). *The urban neighborhood: A sociological perspective.* New York: Random House.

Kelly, R. F. (1982). The family and the analysis of the underclass: An integrative framework. Paper presented to the meeting of the American Society of Criminology.

Kenny, D. A. (1979). *Correlation and causality.* New York: Wiley-Interscience.

Kessler, R. C. & Greenberg, D. F. (1981). *Linear panel analysis.* New York: Academic Press.

Kitagawa, E. M. & Taeuber, K. E., (1963) *Local community fact book. Chicago metropolitan area. 1960.* Chicago: Chicago Community Inventory.

Kleck, G. (1979). Capital punishment, gun ownership and homicide. *American Journal of Sociology 84 (4, January)*, 882–910.

Kleck, G. (1984a). The relationship between gun ownership levels and rates of violence in the United States. In {D. B. Kates, Jr., (Ed.),} *Firearms and violence: Issues of public policy* Pacific Institute for Public Policy Research. New York: Ballinger Publishing Company.

Kleck, G. (1984b). Handgun-Only Gun Control: A Policy Disaster in the Making. In D. B. Kates, Jr., (Ed.), *Firearms and Violence: Issues of Public Policy* Pacific Institute for Public Policy Research. New York: Ballinger Publishing Company.

Kleck, G. & Bordua, D. J. (1984). The assumptions of gun control. In {Don B. Kates, Jr., (Ed.),} *Firearms and violence: Issues of public policy.* Pacific Institute for Public Policy Research. Cambridge: MA: Ballinger Publishing Company.

Kleck, G. & Bordua, D. J. (1983). The factual foundations for certain key assumptions of gun control. *Law and Policy Quarterly 5 (July)*, 271–298.

Kleinbaum, D. & Kupper, L. (1978). *Applied regression analysis and other multivariable methods*. Belmont, CA: Wadsworth.

Kornhauser, R. (1978). *Social sources of delinquency*. Chicago, IL: University of Chicago Press.

Kowalski, C. et al. (1980). Spatial distributions of criminal offenses by states: 1970–76. *Journal of Research in Crime and Delinquency 17*, 4–25.

Krug, A. S. (1968). The relationship between firearms ownership and crime rates. *Congressional Record 114 (January)*, 1496–98.

Krus, D. J., Sherman, J. L. & Krus, P. (1977). Changing values over the last half-century: The story of Thurstone's crime scales. *Psychological Reports 40*, 207–211.

Langbein, L. & Lichtman, A. (1978). *Ecological inference*. Beverly Hills, CA: Sage.

Lander, B. (1954). *Toward an understanding of juvenile delinquency*. New York: Columbia University Press.

Laub, J. H. (1983). *Criminology in the making: An oral history*. Boston: Northeastern University Press.

Laub, J. H. (1980). Criminal behavior and the urban-rural dimension. Ph.D. dissertation. Albany: State University of New York at Albany.

Levin, Y. & Lindesmith, A. (1937). English ecology and criminology of the past century. *Journal of Criminal Law and Criminology 27*, 801–816.

Lewin, K. (1936). *Principles of topological psychology*. New York: McGraw-Hill.

Lewis, D. A. (1981). *Reactions to crime*. Beverly Hills, CA: Sage Publications.

Lewis, D. A. & Salem, G. (1981). Community crime prevention: an analysis of a developing strategy. *Crime and Delinquency 27 (3)*, 405–421.

Lewis, D. A. & Salem, G. (1980). *Crime and urban community: Towards a theory of urban security*. Evanston, IL: Northwestern University, Center for Urban Affairs.

Lewis, O. (1965). The folk-urban ideal types: Further observations on the folk-urban continuum and urbanization with special reference to Mexico City, pp. 491–503 in Hauser and Schnore (Eds.) *The study of urbanization*. New York: Wiley.

Lewis-Beck, M. (1980). *Applied regression: An introduction*. Sage University Paper 22. Beverly Hills, CA: Sage Publications.

Lizotte, A. J. & Bordua, D. J. (1980). Firearms ownership for sport and protection: Two divergent models *American Sociological Reveiw 45 (April)*, 229–244.

Lizotte, A. J., Bordua, D. J., & White, C. S. (1981). Firearms ownership for sport and protection: Two not so divergent models. *American Sociological Review 46 (August)*, 499–503.

Loftin, C. & Hill, R. H. (1974). Regional subculture and homicide: An examination of the Gastil-Hackney thesis. *American Sociological Review 39*, 714–724.

Long, S. K. & Witte, A. D. (1981). Current economic trends: Implications for crime and criminal justice, pp. 69–143 in K. N. Wright (Ed.) *Crime and criminal justice in a declining economy*. Cambridge: Gelgeschlager, Gunn and Hain.

Maccoby, E., Johnson, J., Church, R. (1958). Community integration and the social control of juvenile delinquency. *Journal of Social Issues 14 (3)*, 38–51.

Mann, P. H. (1970). The neighborhood, pp. 568–583 in R. Gutman & D. Popenoe (Eds.), *Neighborhood, city, and metropolis*. New York: Random House.

Mannheim, H. & Wilkins, L. T. (1955). *Prediction methods in relation to Borstal training.* London: Her Majesty's Stationery Office.

Matza, D. (1969). *Becoming deviant.* Englewood Cliffs, NJ: Prentice-Hall.

Matza, D. (1964). *Delinquency and drift.* New York: Wiley.

Mayhew, H. (1862). *London labour and the London poor.* London: Griffin, Bohn.

McCaghy, C. H. (1980). *Crime in American society.* New York: Macmillan Publishing Company, Inc.

McDowall, D. & Loftin, C. (1983). Collective security and the demand for legal handguns. *American Journal of Sociology 88(6),* 1146–1161.

Meehl, P. E. (1954). *Clinical versus statistical prediction.* Minneapolis: University of Minnesota Press.

Meehl, P. E., & Rosen, A. (1955). Antecedent probability and the efficiency of psychometric signs, patterns, or cutting scores. *Psychological Bulletin 52 (3),* 194–216.

Merry, S. E. (1981a). *Urban danger: Life in a neighborhood of strangers.* Philadelphia, PA: Temple University Press.

Merry, S. E. (1981b) Defensible space undefended. *Urban Affairs Quarterly 16 (4),* 397–422.

Merton, R. K. (1957). *Social theory and social structure.* New York: Free Press.

Merton, R. K. (1938). Social structure and anomie. *American Sociological Review 3,* 672–682.

Messner, S. (1983). Regional and racial effects on the urban homicide rate: The subculture of violence revisited. *American Journal of Sociology 88,* 997–1007.

Messner, S. (1982). Poverty, inequality and the urban homicide rate. *Criminology 20,* 103–114.

Michelson, W. H. (1970). *Man and his urban environment: A sociological approach.* Reading, MA: Addison-Wesley.

Mischel, W. (1968). *Personality assessment.* New York: Wiley.

Mitchell, J. C. (1969). Social networks. *Annual Review of Anthropology 3,* 279–299.

Mladenka, P. & Hill, J. (1976). A reexamination of the etiology of urban crime. *Criminology 13 (4),* 491–505.

Monahan, J. (1981). *Predicting violent behavior: An assessment of clinical techniques.* Beverly Hills, CA: Sage.

Monahan, J. & Klassen D. (1982). Situational approaches to understanding and predicting individual violent behavior, pp. 292–319 in M. Wolfgang and N. Weiner (Eds.), *Criminal violence.* Beverly Hills, CA: Sage.

Moore, M. (1983). Controlling criminogenic commodities: Drugs, guns, and alcohol. In J. O. Wilson (Ed.) Crime and public policy. San Francisco: ICS Press.

Morris, T. (1957). *The criminal area: A study in social ecology.* London: Routledge and Kegan Paul.

Murray, C. (1983). The physical environment and community control of crime, pp. 107–124 in J. Q. Wilson (Ed.), *Crime and public policy.* San Francisco, CA: Institute for Contemporary Studies.

Murray, D. R. (1975). "Handguns, gun control laws, and firearms violence." *Social Problems (October),* 81–93.

Myers, S. L., Jr. (1980). Why are crimes underreported? What is the crime rate? Does it *really* matter? *Social Science Quarterly 61, 1 (June)*, 23–43.

Myers, S. L., Jr. (1978). The economics of crime in the urban ghetto. *Reveiw of Black Political Economy 9 (1)*, 43–59.

National Academy of Sciences (1981). *New directions in the rehabilitation of criminal offenders*. Washington, DC: National Academy Press.

Nelson, J. (1980). Multiple victimization in American cities: A statistical analysis of rare events. *American Journal of Sociology 85*, 870–891.

Nelson, J. (1979). Implications for the ecological study of crime, in W. Parsonage (Ed.), *Victimology*. Beverly Hills, CA: Sage.

Nelson, J. (1978). *Similarities and differences in the relationship of personal victimization to demographic variables in 26 American cities*. Albany, NY: Criminal Justice Research Center.

Newman, O. (1972). *Defensible space*. New York: Collier.

Newton, G. D. & Zimring, F. E. (1969). Firearms and violence in american life: A staff report to the National Commission on the Causes and Prevention of Violence. Washington, DC: US Government Printing Office.

O'Brien, R. (1983). Metropolitan structure and violent crime: Which measure of crime? *American Sociological Review 48*, 434–437.

O'Brien, R., Shichor, D., & Becker, D. L. (1980). An empirical comparison of the validity of UCR and NCS crime rates. *Sociological Quarterly 21*, 391–401.

O'Connor, J. F. & Lizotte, A. J. (1978). The Southern subculture of violence thesis and patterns of gun ownership. *Social Problems 25 (April)*, 420–429.

Olweus, D. (1977). A critical analysis of the 'modern' interactionist position, pp. 221–234 in D. Magnusson & N. S. Endler (Eds.), *Personality at the crossroads: Current issues in interactional psychology*. Hillsdale, NJ: Erlbaum.

Orleans, P. (1969). Robert Park and social area analysis, in P. Meadows & E. Mizruchi (Eds.), *Urbanism, urbanization and change: Comparative perspective*. Reading, MA: Addison-Wesley.

Orsagh, T. (1979). Empirical criminology: Interpreting results derived from aggregate data. *Journal of Research in Crime and Delinquency (July)*, 294–306.

Park, R. E. (1916) The city. *American Journal of Sociology 20 (5)*, 577–612.

Parker, R. N. & Smith, M. D. (1979). Deterrence, poverty and type of homicide. *American Journal of Sociology 85*, 614–624.

Pettigrew, T. F. & Spier, R. B. (1962). The ecological structure of negro homicide. *American Journal of Sociology 67 (6)*, 621–629.

Pfohl, E. (1985). *Images of deviance and social control: A sociological history*. New York: McGraw-Hill.

Piven, F. F. & Cloward, R. (1982). *The new class war*. New York: Pantheon.

Piven, F. F. & Cloward, R. (1971). *Regulating the poor*. New York: Random House.

Pokorny, A. (1965). Human violence: A comparison of homicide, aggravated assault, suicide and attempted suicide. *Journal of Criminal Law, Criminology, and Police Science 56*, 488–497.

Polk, K. E. (1967). Urban social areas and delinquency. *Social Problems 14*, 320–325.

Polk, K. E. (1957–1958). Juvenile delinquency and social areas. *Social Problems 5*, 214–217.

Popenoe, D. (1973). Urban residential differentiation: An overview of patterns, trends, and problems. *Sociological Inquiry 43*, 35–56.

Pyle, G. (1974). *The spatial dynamics of crime*. Chicago, IL: University of Chicago Department of Geography.

Quinney, R. (1966). Structural characteristics, population areas, and crime rates in the United States. *Journal of Criminal Law, Criminology and Police Science 57, 1 (January)*, 45–52.

Quinney, R. (1964). Crime, delinquency and social areas. *Journal of Research in Crime and Delinquency 1*, 149–154.

Rainwater, L. (1970). *Behind ghetto walls: Black families in a federal slum*. Chicago, IL: Aldine.

Rawson, R. W. (1839). An inquiry into the statistics of crime in England and Wales. *Journal of the Statistical Society of London, 2*, 316–344.

Reckless, W. C. (1973). *The crime problem*. New York: Appleton-Century-Croft.

Reiss, A. (1967). *Studies in crime and law enforcement in major metropolitan areas*. Volume 1, Section 1: Measurement of the nature and the amount of crime. Field Surveys III. Washington, DC: U.S. Government Printing Office. President's Commission on Law Enforcement and Administration of Justice.

Reiss, A. J. Jr. (1976). Settling the frontiers of a pioneer in American criminology: Henry McKay, pp. 64–90 in J. F Short (Ed.) *Delinquency, crime, and society*. Chicago: University of Chicago Press.

Reiss, A. J. Jr. [Ed.] (1964). On cities and social life: Selected papers. Chicago: University of Chicago Press.

Reiss, A. & Rhodes, A. (1961). The distribution of juvenile delinquency in the social class structure. *American Sociological Review 26*, 720–732.

Reitzes, D. C. (1955). The effect of social environment upon former felons. *Journal of Criminal Law, Criminology, and Police Science 46 (2)*, 226–231.

Rich, W., Sutton, L., Clear, T., & Saks, M. (1982). *Sentencing by mathematics: An evaluation of the early attempts to develop and implement sentencing guidelines*. A publication of the National Center for State Courts.

Riley, D. (1985). Time and crime. Paper presented at the annual meeting of the American Society of Criminology, San Diego, California.

Ritzer, G. (1975). *Sociology: A multiple paradigm science*. Boston, MA: Allyn and Bacon.

Rockwell, R. C. (1975). Assessment of multicollinearity: The Haitovsky test of the determinant. *Sociological Methods and Research 3*, 308–320.

Rohe, W. & Gates, L. (1981). Neighborhood planning: Promise and product. *Urban and Social Change Review 14 (1)*, 26–32.

Roncek, D. (1981). Dangerous places: Crime and residential environment. *Social Forces 60*, 74–96.

Roncek, D. (1975). Density and crime: A methodological critique. *American Behavioral Scientist 18*, 843–861.

Rosen, L. & K. Neilson (1978). The broken home and delinquency, pp. 406–415 in L. Savitz and N. Johnston (Eds.) *Crime in society*. New York: Wiley.

Rosenfeld, R. (1984). Inequality and crime. Ph.D. dissertation. Oregon: University of Oregon, Department of Sociology.

Rosenfeld, R. (1982). "Inequality, relative deprivation and crime: Explaining some discrepant findings. Paper presented at the 1982 annual meeting of the American Society of Criminology, Toronto, Canada.

Rosenfeld, R. (1979). Income inequality and urban crime, pp. 291–319 in G. A. Tobin (Ed.), *The changing structure of the city: What happened to the urban crisis.* Beverly Hills, CA: Sage.

Rossi, P., Waite, E., Bose, C., & Berk, R. (1974). The seriousness of crime: Normative structure and individual differences. *American Sociological Review 39,* 224–237.

Runciman, W. G. (1966). *Relative deprivation and social justice.* Berkeley: University of California Press.

Sagi, P. and Wellford, C. (1968). Age composition and patterns of change in criminal statistics. *Journal of Criminal Law, Criminology and Police Science.*

Sampson, R. (1985). Neighborhood and crime: The structural determinants of personal victimization. *Journal of Research in Crime and Delinquency 22,* 7–40.

Sampson, R. (1983a). Structural density and criminal victimization. *Criminology 21,* 276–293.

Sampson, R. (1983b). Neighborhood context of criminal victimization. Ph.D. dissertation. Albany: State University of New York at Albany.

Sampson, R. & Castellano, T. (1982). Economic inequality and personal victimization: an areal perspective. *British Journal of Criminology 22,* 363–385.

Sampson, R., Castellano, T., & Laub, J. (1981). *Analysis of National Crime Survey Data to study serious delinquent behavior.* Volume 5: Juvenile Criminal Behavior and Its Relation to Neighborhood Characteristics. Washington, DC: U.S. Government Printing Office.

Savitz, L. (1978). Official police statistics and their limitations. In L. Savitz and N. Johnson (Eds.) *Crime in society.* New York: Wiley

Savitz, L. (1970). Delinquency and migration. In L. Savitz and N. Johnson (Eds.) *Crime in society.* New York: Wiley.

Schlossman, S., Zellman, G., Shavelson, R., Sedlak, M., & Cobb, J. (1984). Delinquency prevention in South Chicago: *A fifty year assessment of the Chicago Area Project.* Santa Monica, CA: Rand Corporation.

Schmid, C. F. (1960). Urban crime areas. *American Sociological Review 25,* 537–542 (Part I); 655–678 (Part II).

Schmidt, P. & Witte, A. (1979). Models of criminal recidivism and an illustration of their use in evaluating correctional programs, pp. 210–224 in National Research Council, Panel on Research on Rehabilitation Techniques, *The rehabilitation of criminal offenders.* Washington, DC: National Academy of Sciences.

Schuerman, L. A. & Kobrin, S. (1983). Crime and urban ecological processes: Implications for public policy. Paper presented to the Annual Meeting of the American Society of Criminology, Denver, Colorado.

Schuessler, K. F. (1962). Components of variations in city crime rates. *Social Problems 9,* 314–323.

Schur, E. (1971). *Labeling deviant behavior.* New York: Harper and Row.

Sellin, T. & Wolfgang, M. (1964). *The measurement of delinquency.* New York: Wiley.

Shah, S. A. (1978). Dangerousness: A paradigm for exploring some issues in law and psychology. *American Psychologist 33,* 224–238.

Shaw, C. & McKay, H. (1942). *Juvenile delinquency and urban areas.* Chicago, IL: University of Chicago Press.

Shaw, C. & McKay, H. (1931). *Social factors in juvenile delinquency.* Volume 2 of the

Report on the Causes of Crime. National Commission of Law Observance and Enforcement. Washington DC: U.S. Government Printing Office.

Shaw, C. & McKay, H. (1929). *Delinquency areas.* Chicago, IL: University of Chicago Press.

Shevky, E. & Bell, W. (1955). *Social area analysis: Theory, illustrative applications, and computational procedures.* Stanford: Stanford University Press.

Shichor, D., Decker, D. L., & O'Brien, R. M. (1980). The relationship of criminal victimization, police per capita and population density in twenty-six cities. *Journal of Criminal Justice 8*, 309–316.

Shichor, D., Decker, D. L., & O'Brien, R. M. (1979). Population density and criminal victimization: Some unexpected findings in central cities. *Criminology 17, 2 (August)*, 184–193.

Short, J. F. (1979). On the etiology of delinquent behavior. *Journal of Research in Crime and Delinquency (January)*, 28–33.

Short, J. F. [Ed.] (1976). *Delinquency, crime, and society.* Chicago: University of Chicago Press.

Shrout, P. E. & Fleiss, J. L. (1979). Intraclass correlations: Uses in assessing rater reliability. *Psychological Bulletin 86*, 420–2427.

Shumaker, S. A. & Taylor, R. B. (1983). Toward a clarification of people-place relationships: A model of attachment to place, pp. 219–251 in N. R. Feimer & E. S. Geller (Eds.), *Environmental psychology: Directions and perspectives.* New York: Praeger.

Silberman, C. E. (1978). *Criminal violence, criminal justice.* New York: Random House.

Simcha-Fagan, O., & Sampson, R. (1983). Delinquency in environmental context. Working paper, Columbia Univeristy.

Simon, F. H. (1971). *Prediction methods in criminology.* London: Her Majesty's Stationery Office.

Skogan, W. (1986). Fear of crime and neighborhood change. In A. J. Reiss, Jr. M. Tonry (Eds.), *Communities and crime* (special edition of Crime and justice.) Chicago: University of Chicago Press, in press.

Skogan, W. (1979). Crime in contemporary America, pp. 375–391 in H. D. Graham & T. R. Gurr (Eds.), *Violence in America: Historical and comparative perspectives* (revised edition). Beverly Hills, CA: Sage.

Skogan, W. (1975). Measurement problems in official and survey crime rates. *Journal of Criminal Justice 3*, 17–32.

Skogan, W. & Maxfield, M. G. (1981). Coping with crime: individual and neighborhood reactions. Beverly Hills, CA: Sage.

Skogan, W. & Maxfield, M. G. (1980). *The reactions to crime papers.* Vol. I. Coping with crime: Victimization, fear, and reactions to crime in three American cities. Evanston, IL: Northwestern Univeristy, Center for Urban Affairs.

Smith, M. P. (1979). *The city and social theory.* New York: St. Martin's Press.

Snodgrass, J. (1976). Clifford R. Shaw and Henry D. McKay: Chicago criminologists. *British Journal of Criminology 16*, 1–19.

Solomon, H. (1976). Parole outcome: A multidimensional contingency table analysis. *Journal of Research in Crime and Delinquency 13*, 107–126.

Sorensen, A. & Taeuber, K. (1975). Indexes of residential segregation for 109 cities in the U.S., 1940–1970. *Sociological Focus 8*, 125–142.

Sparks, R. (1981). Criminal opportunities and crime rates, pp. 18–28 in S.

Fienberg and A. J. Reiss (Eds.), *Indicators of crime and criminal justice: Qualitative studies*. Washington, DC: U.S. Government Printing Office.

Sparks, R. F., Glenn, H. G. & Dodd, D. J. (1977). *Surveying victims: A study of the measurement of criminal victimization*. New York: John Wiley and Sons.

Sparks, R. F., Greer, A., & Manning, S. (1982). *Theoretical studies*. Final Report, Center for the Study of the Causes of Crime for Gain, School for Criminal Justice, Rutgers University, Newark, New Jersey.

Spergel, I. (1964). *Racketville, slumtown, haulberg*. Chicago: University of Chicago Press.

Stafford, M. C. & Gibbs, J. P. (1980). Crime rates in an ecological context: Extension of a propostion. *Social Science Quarterly 61, 3, 4 (December)*, 653–665.

Stahura, J. M., Huff, C. R. & Smith, B. L. (1978). Crime in the suburbs: A structural model. Paper prepared for presentation at the 73rd Annual Meeting of the American Sociological Association, September 4–8, San Francisco.

Stark, R., Bainbridge, W., Crutchfield, R., Doyle, D., & Finke, R. (1983). Crime and delinquency in the roaring twenties. *Journal of Research in Crime and Delinquency 20*, 4–23.

Stark, R., Kent, L., Doyle, D. (1982). Religion and delinquency: the ecology of a 'lost' relationship. *Journal of Research in Crime and Delinquency 18*, 4–24.

Stokols, D. (1972). On the distinction between density and crowding. *Psychological Review 79*, 275–277.

Stollmack, S. & Harris, C. M. Failure rate analysis applied to recidivism data. *Operations Research 22*, 1192–1205.

Strauss, M. A. (1980). *Behind closed doors*. Garden City, NY: Anchor.

Sutherland, E. & Cressey, D. R. (1974). *Principles of criminology*. Philadelphia: Lippincott.

Suttles, G. D. (1972). *The social construction of communities*. Chicago: University of Chicago Press.

Suttles, G. D. (1968). The social order of the slum. Chicago: University of Chicago Press.

Taub, R. P., Taylor, D. G., Dunham, J. D. (1984). *Paths of neighborhood change: Race and crime in urban America*. Chicago: University of Chicago Press.

Taub, R. P., Taylor, D. G., Dunham, J. D., (1981). Neighborhoods and safety, pp. 103–119 in D. A. Lewis (Ed.), *Reactions to crime*. Beverly Hills, CA: Sage.

Taylor, R. B. (in press). Toward an environmental psychology of disorder, in I. Altman and D. Stokols (Eds.) *Neighborhood environmental psychology*. New York: Wiley.

Taylor, R. B. (1982). Neighborhood physical environment and stress, pp. 286–324 in G. W. Evans (Ed.), *Environmental stress*. New York: Cambridge University Press.

Taylor, R. B., Brower, S., Drain, W. (1979). *Toward a neighborhood-based data file*. Baltimore, MD: Center for Metropolitan Planning and Research, The Johns Hopkins University.

Taylor, R. B. & Gottfredson, S. D. (1983). *The correctional crisis: Prison populations and public policy*. Washington, DC: U.S. Department of Justice.

Taylor, R. B., Gottfredson, S. D., Brower, S. (1980). The defensibility of defensible space, pp. 53–71 in T. Hirschi & M. Gottfredson (Eds.), *Understanding crime*. Beverly Hills, CA: Sage.

Taylor, R. B., Shumaker, S. A., & Gottfredson, S. D. (1985). Neighborhood-level links between physical features and legal sentiments; Deterioration, fear of crime, and confidence. *Journal of Arachitectural Research and Planning, Research* 2, 261-275.

Taylor, R. B. & Talalay, R. (1981). *A decade of population change in Baltimore neighborhoods: Census Note 2.* Baltimore, MD: Center for Metropolitan Planning and Research, The Johns Hopkins University.

Thompson, J. W., Sviridoff, M. & McElroy, J. E. (1981). *Employment and crime: A review of theories and research.* Washington, DC: National Institute of Justice.

Thrasher, .F. M. (1927). *The gang: A study of 1,313 gangs in Chicago.* Chicago: University of Chicago Press.

Thurstone, L. L. (1927). The method of paired comparisons for social values. *Journal of Abnormal and Social Psychology 21*, 384-400.

Tomeh, A., (1973). Formal voluntary organizations: Participation, Correlates, and interrelationships. *Sociological Inquiry 43*, 89-121.

Tomeh, A. (1964). Informal group praticipation and residential patterns. *American Journal of Sociology 70*, 28-35.

Tonso, W. R. (1984). Social problems and sagecraft: Gun control as a case in point. In {D. B. Kates, Jr., (Ed.),} *Firearms and violence: Issues of public policy* Pacific Institute for Public Policy Research. Cambridge, MA: Ballinger Publishing Company.

Turnbull, B. (1977). Note on the non-parametric analysis of the Stollmack-Harris recidivism data. *Operations Research 25*, 706-708.

Underwood, B. (1970) Law and the crystal ball: Predicting behavior with statistical inference and individualized judgement. *Yale Law Journal 88 (6)*, 1408-1448.

U.S. Bureau of the Census (1983a) *Census of population and housing, 1980; County population by age, sex, race, and spanish origin (Preliminary OMB-consistent modified race).* Tape Technical Documentation. Washington, D.C.: Data Users Service Division.

U.S. Bureau of the Census (1983b) Census race data for counties meet OMB criteria. *Data Users News, Vol. 18, No. 9 (September)*, 9.

U.S. Bureau of the Census. (1982). *1980 Census of Population. Vol. I Characteristics of the Population.* Washington, D. C.: PC 80-1 U.S. Government Printing Office.

U.S. Bureau of the Census (1978). *The social and economic status of the black poplation in the United States: An historical view 1790-1978.* Current Population Reports Special Studies Series P-23 No. 80. (1973) *U.S. Census of population: 1970). Vol. I. Characteristics of the population.* Washington, DC: U.S. Government Printing Office.

U.S. Bureau of the Census. (1963). *U.S. Census of population: 1960.* Vol. I. Characteristics of the population. Washington, D.C.: U.S. Government Printing Office.

U.S. Bureau of the Census (Undated) *Public use samples of basic records from the 1970 census: Description and technial documentation.* Technical Report 1. Office of Management and Budget.

U.S. Department of Commerce, Bureau of Census (1977). *County and city data book (A statistical abstract supplement).* Washington, DC: U.S. Government Printing Office.

U.S. President's Commission on Law Enforcement and Administration of Justice

(1967). *Task force report: Crime and its impact—An assessment.* Washington, DC: U.S. Government Printing Office.

Van Alstyne, D. & Gottfredson, M. R. (1978). A multidimensional contingency table analysis of parole outcome. *Journal of Research in Crime and Delinquency 15*, 172–193.

Van Valey, T. J., Roof, W. C., & Wilcox, J. E. (1976). Trends in residental segregation: 1960–1970. *American Journal of Sociology 82 (4)*, 826–844.

Vold, T. (1958). *Theoretical criminology.* New York: Oxford University Press.

Waldo, G. & Griswold D. (1979). Issues in the measurement of recidivism, pp. 225–250 in National Research Council, Panel of Research on Rehabilitation Techniques, *The Rehabilitation of Criminal Offenders.* Washington, DC: National Academy of Sciences.

Walker, S. (1985). *Sense and nonsense about crime.* Monterey, CA: Brooks/Cole Publishing.

Walton, J. & Carns, D. C. (1973). *Cities in change: Studies in the urban condition.* Boston: Allyn and Bacon, Inc.

Wandersman, A. & Florin, P. (1981). A cognitive social learning approach to the cross-roads of cognition, social behavior, and environment, in J. H. Harvey (Ed.), *Cognition, social behavior, and the environment.* Hillsdale, NJ: Erlbaum.

Warren, D. I. (1978). Explorations in neighborhood differentiation. *Sociological Quarterly 19*, 310–331.

Warren, D. I. (1977). The functional diversity of urban neighborhoods. *Urban Affairs Quarterly 13*, 151–180.

Warren. D. I. (1969). Neighborhood structure and riot behavior in Detroit. *Social Problems 16*, 464–484.

Warren, R. L. (1963). *The community in America.* Chicago: Rand McNally.

Watts, A. D. & Watts, T. W. (1981). Minorities and urban crime. *Urban Affairs Quarterly 16*, 423–436.

Webb, S. D. (1972). Crime and the division of labor: Testing a Durkeimian model. *American Journal of Sociology 78 (3)*, 643–656.

Webster, W. (1978). *Crime in the United States, 1977.* Washington, DC: U.S. Government Printing Office.

Wellman, B. & Leighton, B. (1979). Neighborhoods, networks, and communities: Approaches to the study of the community question. *Urban Affairs Quarterly 14*, 363–390.

Whyte, W. F. (1955). *Street corner society.* Chicago: University of Chicago Press.

Wilbanks, W. & Hindelang, M. (1972). The comparative efficiency of three predictive methods, Appendix B in D. M. Gottfredson, L. T. Wilkins, & P. B. Hoffman (Eds.), *Summarizing experience for parole decision-making.* Davis, CA: National Council on Crime and Delinqucy Research Center.

Wilkinson, K. (1980). The broken home and delinquency. In T. Hirschi & M. Gottfredson (Eds.), *Understanding crime.* Beverly Hills, CA: Sage.

Williams, K. (1984). Economic Sources of Homicide: Re-estimating the effect of poverty and inequality. *American Sociological Review 49*, 283–289.

Willie, C. V. (1967). The relative contribution of family status and economic status to juvenile delinquency. *Social Problems 14*, 326–335.

Wilson, J. Q. (1975). *Thinking about crime.* New York: Basic Books.

Wilson, J. Q. [Ed.] (1983) *Crime and public policy.* San Francisco, CA: Institute for Contemporary Studies Press.

Wilson, W. J. (1980). *The declining significance of race: Blacks and changing american institutions (2nd ed.).* Chicago: University of Chicago Press.

Wilson, W. J. & K. Neckerman. (1985). Poverty and family structure: The widening gap between evidence and public policy issues. Paper presented at the conference on Poverty and Policy: Retrospect and Prospects. Williamsburg, Virginia.

Wirth, L. (1964). *On cities and social life: Selected papers.* A. J. Reiss (Ed.). Chicago: University of Chicago Press.

Wirth, L. (1938). Urbanism as a way of life. *American Journal of Sciology 44 (July)*, 1–24.

Wolfgang, M. & Ferracuti, F. (1967). *The subculture of violence: Toward an integrated theory in criminology.* London: Tavistock.

Wright, J. D. & Marston, L. (1975). The ownership of the means of destruction: Weapons in the United States. *Social Problems 23 (1, October)*, 93–107.

Wright, J. D., Rossi, P. H., & Daly, K. (1983). *Under the gun: Weapons, crime and violence in America.* New York: Aldine Publishing Company.

Zimring, F. E. (1968). Is gun control likely to reduce violent killings? *University of Chicago Law Review 35 (Summer)* 721–37.

Zimring, F. E. (1981). "Kids, groups, and crime: Some implications of a well known secret. *Journal of Criminal Law and Criminology 72*, 867–885.

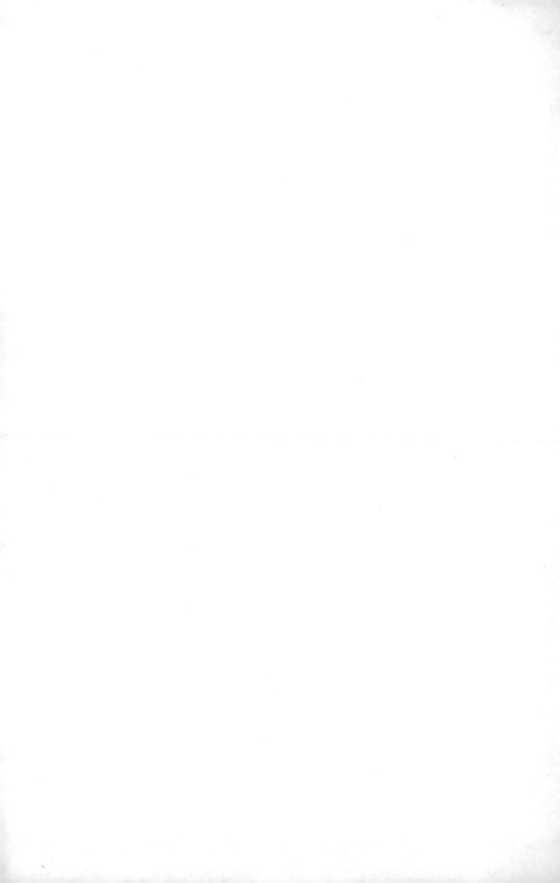

Author Index

Subject Index

Note: The letter N following a page number indicates that the information is contained in the footnote.